YTTC 200 Hrs Students' Manual

By Kavita Sinha

Table of Contents

WELCOME NOTE

Creation has been made by the love of the divine consciousness and yoga makes life rejoice in this love. It is known that overall health is signified not just by the absence of disease, but also denotes being healthy emotionally and physically. WHO also has suggested a fourth dimension which is 'spiritual wellbeing". Good health hence denotes; by a combination of

1. Good body health - Average height and weight; with the absence of any disease. The essential factors to maintain physical health are regular exercise, proper diet and nutrition and proper relaxation or rest for recovering or rejuvenation.

2. Mental and social health - Good cognitive and emotional well - being is having good mental health and this is more of a subjective assessment. . Social wellbeing is having an ability to make a contribution to one's community and to work productively and fruitfully.

3. Spiritual wellbeing - Today's modern and industrial world has made us encounter a lot of pollution and infections and has also

resulted in an unnatural and/or faulty lifestyle that causes stress. Moreover, unhealthy dietary habits like eating preserved foods, high calorie foods, smoking, drinking, drugs and lack of exercise induces stress and related psychosomatic diseases like diabetes, high blood pressure, arthritis, back pain and so on. In this scenario, spiritual well - being can help in combating all the challenges of modernization.

In this context, yoga promotes physical and psychological wellbeing, improves efficiency and productivity and improves the lifestyle. Knowing about the techniques and practice of yoga is made possible in this course.

This yoga manual will help you to learn yoga theory and practice and has been written keeping in view the practical aspects of yoga practice. The manual is meant for yoga teachers for their YTTC course.

They can distribute a copy to their students as their

course book.

Have a happy and successful yoga learning and
teaching practice.

Peace, health and happiness!!

Kavita and Team

PRAYERS AND INTRODUCTION TO YOGA

Starting and completing a yoga practice with prayers is expected, as it connects you within yourself and connects you with the sounds of prayers. It enables you to practice yoga in a relaxed manner as it is meant to be.

Prayers can be said in any language and any form. Om chanting is a practice at the beginning and completion of any yoga practice. 'Om' in Christianity and Islam it is called "Amen", in Jewish religion it is called 'Shalom' and in the Sikh, Jain and Hindu religions it is called "Om".

Science has confirmed that sound is a form of energy and even the universe started with a big bang. Therefore, chanting prayers harnesses the energy of sound within you and helps you to remain calm, rested, peaceful and aware of the surrounding and of the life force within you. Prayers can also reduce the pain and sorrows of life.

Yogic Prayer

1. Sit easily and comfortably with eyes gently closed and hands in Prayer or Anjali Mudra

2. Relax your shoulders and relax your whole body and take 2 - 5 long and deep breaths

3. Chant 'AUM" 3 times, keeping the sound of 'AU' and 'M' of equal length.

4. Invoke the Agni fire by rubbing your palms together until they are warm feeling the activation of energy within you

5. Place the palms over the eyes very gently, feeling happiness and lightness

6. Then very slowly open your eyes and look at your palms

You are now ready for your yoga practice

SLOKA BEFORE YOGA PRACTICE

1) Evocation to the sage Patanjali

"YOGENA CHITTASYA PADENA VACHA

MALAM SHARIRASYA KA VAIDYAKENA

YO PAAKARO TTAMAM PRAVARAM MUNINAM

PATANJALIM PRAAN JALIR - ANATO ASMI

ABAHU PURUSHAKARAM;

SHANKA CHAKRASI DHARINAM

SAHASRA SIRASAM SVETAM,

PRANAMAMI PATANJALIM

OM, SHANTI, SHANTI, SHANTIHI"

Meaning

Through Yoga the Chitra, through Grammar the

Language

And through medicine the physical body

Among all those Sages who handed this over

I respectfully bow to Patanjali

The upper body of the human shape carrying a

mussel horn (original tone) a discus (infinity) and a

sword (power of differentiation)

Having 1000 bright heads, I bow to Patanjali

Om Peace, Peace, Peace

(2)   "OM SAHANA VAVATHU, SAHANAU

BHUNAKTU

SAHA VEERYAM KARAVA HAI

TEJASWI NA VADHITAMASTU

MA VIDWISHAVAHAI

OM SHANTI, SHANTI, SHANTIHI "

Meaning:

"Oh Lord! Protect all of us and help all of us

That we get capacity to study and understand (the

scriptures)

With the acquisition of this knowledge, let peace

flow in us

Help us to become brilliant

To not hold any grudges (enmity) against anyone

Om, Peace! Peace! Peace!"

SLOKA AFTER YOGA PRACTICE

   (1)"OM SARVE BHAVANTU SUKHINAH

SARVE SANTU NIRAAMAYAAH

SARVE BHADRANI PASHYANTU

MA KASCHID DUKHA BHAG BHAVET

OM SHANTI, SHANTI, SHANTIHI"

Meaning

"Oh Lord! May all be happy!

May all be free from diseases!

May all have peace and happiness in their lives!

And no one suffers from sorrows!

Om Peace! Peace! Peace!"

(2)"OM, ASATO MAA SADH GAMAYA

TAMASO MAA JYOTIR GAMAYA

MRITYOR MA AMRITAM GAMAYA

OM SHANTI, SHANTI, SHANTIHI"

Meaning

"Lead me from the unreal to the real

From darkness (ignorance) to light (knowledge)

And from death to immortality

Om Peace! Peace! Peace!

So, you can choose any saying or prayer in any language. The above prayers are an example and you can choose your own prayer also. You can go in for affirmations like "I am healthy", I am peaceful" and "I am calm and happy".

Brief introduction to yoga

Yoga, which has its origins in the Vedas, the oldest record of Indian culture, is an ancient Indian science. Yoga provides a path towards realizing super consciousness beyond sensory perceptions. Yoga deals with the physical, mental, moral and spiritual aspects. It was systematized by the Great Indian sage, Patanjali, in the 'Yoga Sutras' in 900 BC.

We can interpret Yoga from the root word 'yuj' meaning 'to come together'; 'to unite'; 'uniting the individual consciousness with the universal consciousness'.

YOGAH CHITTA VRITTI NIRODHAH' - Yoga is to gain control of the mind by cessation of the modifications of the mind.

'TADA DRASHTUH SWARUPE AVASTHANAM' -

By controlling the modifications of the mind, one can reach the original state

We look deeper inside ourselves, develop the power of concentration and focus in the mind as we learn about yoga.

Techniques of yoga according to Swami Vivekananda

The evolution of life through yoga can be achieved by

- Karma Yoga - The path of karma yoga is to do work or action with a sense of detachment to the fruits of action.

  'Samatvam Yogah Ucyate' - Smatva is 'balanced state' and ucyate means 'said to be' So Karma Yoga brings steadiness in the mind of the practitioner by making the actions and processes as or more important than the results. Karma Yoga cleanses the

- ☐ Instruments of action or 'karmendriyas' and

  ☐ Instruments of understanding or ' jnanendriyas'

- Bhakti Yoga - By totally surrendering through worship and with pure love to the divine, an individual can find the key to the control of emotions. This is very important in the modern age when a person can witness emotions tossing them in all directions. Bhakti Yoga is a very pleasant and practical way of gaining control of emotional instabilities and properly harness the emotional energies

- Jnana Yoga - The Upanishads provide knowledge and rational understanding of 'happiness' and this is the pathway of 'Jnana Yoga'. This is apt for keen individuals. Through the knowledge pathway, Jnana Yoga answers many fundamental questions about the intellect and its basis. In the present age of science, mankind is a rational and logical minded being. Jnana Yoga has importance in the imminence of intellectual sharpness in present days.

- Raja Yoga - Raja Yoga centers on practices that bring about a 'mind culture or psychic control'. Raja Yoga provides a pathway towards success in almost all aspects and endeavors in the practitioner's life. Raja Yoga is a flexible and versatile approach to reaching the higher states of consciousness. Raja Yoga includes all the activities of life as part of its basis. Raja Yoga is based on Patanjali's Ashtanga Yoga system. Ashtanga Yoga is the Eight limbs of Yoga which are:

Yama, Niyama, Asana, Pranayama, Pratyahara, Dharana, Dhyana and Samadhi.

Yoga Practice

The main philosophy of yoga is that mind, body and spirit are one and cannot be clearly separated

The main 5 principles of yoga philosophy

- ANUSHASAN (Discipline): Yogic discipline is not becoming a victim to one's mind, ego and our surroundings and situations. This enables us to manage stress and tensions and to have less complaints and more mindfulness.

- ABHYAS (Practice): Regular and well balanced asana practice, regular breathing exercises, complete relaxation, a healthy diet, self-reflection and positivity. There are less complaints and expectations about the goal and more practice.

- SAMARPAN (Surrender): There is a total surrender of the 'self', unconditional presence, listening and following the guidance provided by the teacher. This unconditional 'samarpan' leads to easy learning and excellent results.

- SHRADDHA (Trust): As a mother cares for and protects her children and draws them away from the dangers of silly whims and fancies, so does the Guru to their students. A Guru is like a family or friend to the student. New learning and knowledge in their lives require the unconditional trust of the Guru by the student.

- VAIRAGYA (Detachment or being in the present moment): Learning something new or teaching others requires detachment from existing perception, likes and dislikes. This type of mindfulness; being in the present moment, and detachment can lead towards excellent results.

The Yoga Sutras

The Yoga Sutras by Patanjali is a collection of 196 short verses within 4 chapters estimated to have been written roughly around 400 CE. The book is regarded as the basis of Yoga philosophy and also as a guide to attain wisdom and self-realization through Yoga.

Yoga Sutras are divided into four chapters:

- I - Samadhi Pada – 51 Sutras

- II – Sadhana Pada – 55 Sutras

- III – Vibhuti Pada – 56 Sutras

- IV – Kaivalya Pada – 34 Sutras

- **Chapter 1: Samadhi Pada – 51 Sutras**

The first sutra begins by giving the instructions on the practice of Yoga

Atha Yoga anushasanam (I – 1)

Atha means 'now' and anushasanam means 'discipline'

So the meaning is "Now is the discipline of yoga".

The second sutra is the definition of Yoga.

Yogaha chitta vritti nirodhah (I – 2)

Chitta means' mind', vritti means' modifications of mind' and nirodhah means 'to control'

Yoga is to control the modifications or fluctuations of the mind.

The third Sutra is about the ultimate achievement of Yoga.

Tada drashtuh swarupe awasthanam (I – 3)

Tada means - 'after that', drashtuh means – 'the seer', swarupe means – 'state of self or soul' and awasthanam means - 'resides'

After that (control of functioning of mind) the seer establishes himself into true state of being

In the first chapter; Samadhi pada, Patanjali explains five types of *vrittis* (types of

modifications of mind). These fluctuations of our mind affect our outer consciousness. They are:

- Pramana or correct knowledge

- Viparyaya or incorrect knowledge, incorrect perception misconception

- Vikalpa: Imagination or fantasy

- Nidra: Sleep

- Smriti: Memory

In the first chapter; Samadhi pada, Patanjali talks about the paths to achieve the goal of mind control.

- One of these is Aumkar chanting.

- Practicing or Abhyasa, that includes simple practices like observing without logic and/or judgement and relaxing

- Different types of *Samadhi* (ultimate state of achievement in yoga) through the path of Bhakti, a complete surrender to God or Ishwara

- Overcoming the 5 types of fluctuations of the mind as mentioned above

- Concentrating and focusing the mind on one task or goal at a time can bring calmness to the mind and natural control over the mind

- **Chapter 2: Sadhana Pada - 55 Sutras**

This chapter focuses on the practices (Sadhanas), the obstacles (kleshas) in the practice, the outcome and fruits of the practice

All eight parts of Ashtanga yoga provide practical guidance and are explained by Patanjali in the last part of the chapter. These are steps or paths of Raja Yoga. They are:

1. Yama – Social Discipline

2. Niyama – Self Discipline

3. Asana – Yoga poses

4. Pranayama – Breath control

5. Pratyahara – Sense withdrawal

6. Dharana – Concentration

7. Dhyana – Meditation and

8. Samadhi – Self-realization

The 5 'kleshas' or obstacles for not attaining the potential of yoga in union with the divine Ishwara are:

- Avidya - Ignorance

- Asmitha - The 'I' feeling or egoism

- Raga - Attachment or passion

- Dvesha - Anger or aversion

- Abhinivesha - becoming attached and clinging to life

- **Chapter 3: Vibhuti Pada – 56 Sutras**

Chapter 3 clarifies the last 2 limbs of yoga being

1. Dhyana – meditation and

2. Samadhi – self-realization

All three together (Dharana, Dhyana and Samadhi) are called Samyama. They are simultaneous practices and Samyama on different objects leads to different achievements which are called Siddhis (perfections) and supernormal abilities are subject to the practice of Samyama.

The final part of the chapter analyzes the empowering of the mind.

- **Chapter 4: Kaivalya Pada – 34 Sutras**

The fourth chapter clarifies the issue of liberation or 'Kaivalya' and how this could be achieved by the mind. 'Vasanas' are also known as 'Samskaras' which are subtle impressions latent in the mind and have karmic effects. They accumulate and give rise to 'Abhinivesha'; which is generally 'a will to live' or 'fear of death' which is expressed as;

  - Feeling uncertain about one's life

- Being afraid of what people think of you

- Not wanting to grow old

- Not wanting to acknowledge your children growing up

- And the like

Abhinivesha is considered as a 'klesha' or obstacle. This klesha is considered to be the deepest and the most universal of all the kleshas.

Vasanas or Samskaras can disappear with the elimination of four factors:

- Hetu - 'cause'

- Phala - 'effect'

- Ashraya - 'support of an experience'

- Alabama - 'object of an experience'

Reorientation oneself into something else deeper and more permanent can help overcome abhinivesha and become enlightened.

In this context is Sutra 11 identifies how the higher mind can help overcome abhinivesha:

'Citta ('higher mind) becomes pure and capable of reflecting both

- The drashta ('observer/ witness') and
- The drishya ('what is seen/ observed').

This chapter ends in sutra 34 by defining liberation (kaivalya) itself:

- "Kaivalya is that state in which Gunas ('qualities') merge in their cause in relation to Purusha ('Pure Consciousness'). In this manner, the Soul becomes established in its true nature, which is Pure Consciousness.

- 'Janmaushadhimantratapaha samadhijah sidhayaha' (IV – 1) explains ways to achieve ultimate state of Samadhi

1. By birth, which are family discipline practices

2. Mantra chanting

3. Practicing Tapa (Austerity)

4. Practice of Yoga

Patanjali's 8 Limbs of Ashtanga Yoga

The 8 parts of the self-discipline of yoga is also known as 'Ashtanga Yoga'. They are divided into

- Bahiranga (Yama, Niyama, Asana, Pranayama, Prathyahara) and
- Antaranga yoga (Dharana, Dhyana, Samadhi)

BAHIRANGA YOGA: Yama, Niyama, Asana, Pranayama, Prathyahara

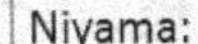

Yama	Niyama:
1.Ahimsa:Non Harming	1. Saucha: Clarity of thoughts and cleanliness of home and surroundings
2. Satya: Benevolence; truthfullness	2. Santosha: Contentment
3. Asteya: Being responsibe to others; Non stealing	3.Tapas: Discipline and sacrifice for others
4. Bhramacharya: Moderation	4. Svadhyaya: Self study
5. Aparigraha: Simplicicty and non-hoarding of things and emotions	5. Ishvara pranidhana: Surrender, bigger service to anything that nature provides

- Yamas - These provide us with what to avoid and self-restraints which paves the way to increase the power of concentration, pure mental state and steadiness of being. The 5 Yamas are

    1. Ahimsa - Nonviolence toward self and others

    2. Satya - To be truthful in thoughts and action toward oneself and others

    3. Asteya - Not to steal tangibles and intangibles from oneself and from others

    4. Brahmacharya - Celibacy and balance of thoughts and deeds

    5. Aparigraha - Not to possess beyond one's actual needs

- Niyamas - Disciplines or fixed observances provide us with the means to attain a gainful and happy life. The 5 Niyamas are

    1. Soucha - Purification and cleanliness (a) Internally within oneself by being mindful

of thoughts, food habits and so on (b)
Externally by keeping our house and
surroundings neat and clean

2. Santosha - Contentment with all things
within oneself and with one's life
achievements

3. Swadhyaya - To acquire correct
knowledge of the self and the supreme
divinity and to study authentic texts and
religious scriptures

4. Ishwar Pranidhan - Complete self-
surrender to the divine will

- Asanas - Postures which are categorized as
special patterns that stabilize the mind and
body through static stretching. The function
isn't simply physical but psycho - neuro
physical. The aim of asanas is to enable
proper mechanisms in the neuromuscular
tonic impulses and improve the tissue, fascia

and muscle tone. The basic principles of asanas are:

- 'Sthira Sukham Asanam' : The posture should be steady and comfortable

- 'Prayatna saithily ananta samapatti bhayam' : The posture is mastered by relaxation of effort and meditation on the endless infinity

- 'Tato dvan dvan nabhig hatah': There should be no jerks and performance of asanas should not lead to fatigue

Classification of asanas

1. Meditative - Meditative asanas are sitting postures. The practitioner sits comfortably, steadily and easily while keeping the head, neck and trunk straight and erect. Meditative asanas include Siddhasana, Swastikasana (auspicious pose), Padmasana, Vajrasana, Muktasana and Sukhasana.

2. Cultural - Cultural asanas involve the whole body. They are almost countless in number and keep the spine flexible. They build up the strength in the back and spinal muscles. They also stimulate proper functioning in the thoracic and abdominal vital organs. As they are asanas, they involve static stretching and help tone up the whole body muscles. Giving two examples in each position, cultural asanas include Pavan Muktasana and Naukasana in the lying down supine position; Bhujangasana and Dhanurasana in the lying down prone position, Paschimmotanasana and Purvatasana in the sitting down position; Namanasana and Hastotanasana in the standing position.

3. Relaxative - Relaxative asanas provide rest and rejuvenation to the body and

mind. They are fewer in number and include Balasana and other poses in the lying down position like Shavasana and Makarasana.

- Pranayama - Pranayama is the regulation of breath. Pranayama helps control the prana, the breath or life force and must be practiced after learning the asanas. The components of breaking are Inhalation (Puraka), Exhalation (Rechaka) and Holding the breath (Kumbhaka). Kumbhaka can be stopping the breath after inhalation (Antara Kumbhaka) and holding the breath after the exhalation (Bahya Kumbhaka). The aim of pranayama is 'Kevala Kumbhaka' which denotes the natural cessation of breath without any conscious effort.

There are many advantages to practicing Pranayama. While energizing the whole body, pranayama also develops deep relaxation and improves metabolic rate. On the spiritual level, Pranayama acts as a mediator between the mind and body giving control over thought processes; a feeling of bliss and expansiveness .Pranayama can be classified as

Cooling Pranayama - Sheetali, Shitkari

Heating Pranayama - Suryabhedana, Bhastrika, Agnisara

Balancing Pranayama - Ujjayi, Anulom Vilom

Calming and Restorative Pranayama - Bhramari, Yogic Breathing

- Pratyahara - Pratyahara is the enabling of the mind from external perceptions and sensory stimuli into the mind and involves introspections and abstractions. Pratyahara is practiced simply by in - drawing of the senses. In - drawing of the senses is done by observing the changes happening within the body and can also be done with the eyes closed if required.

Prathyahara during asana and pranayama practice helps to relax and gain control over the sense organs. It also helps in controlling thought processes by enabling single thought. Therefore, Pratyahara gives the advantage to practice meditation with ease.

ANTARANGA YOGA: Dharana, Dhyana, Samadhi

- Dharana - Dharana is the concentration of the mind on a mantra or object in an uninterrupted flow in contemplation. This mantra or object is also chosen for meditation.

- Dhyana - Dhyana is the relaxed dwelling of the mind on a single thought, mantra or object as the object of meditation.

- Samadhi - Samadhi is a 'super – conscious state' as a result of longer and regular practice of dhyana that leads to a thoughtless state.

Samadhi occurs when there is dhyana or relaxed dwelling in meditation without dwelling on the mind itself.

INTEGRATED APPROACH IN YOGA - THE KOSHAS

Should we always begin yoga on the physical level? There is no prescribed journey and where we begin depends on our personal interest and gradually the interest in one path leads to another. So we can begin yoga with the practice of reading the yoga sutras or by meditation. We can simply begin by practicing asanas, yoga experience of the body or Pranayama, feeling the breath as the movement of our inner being.

An integrated approach to yoga combines the practices with the 'Koshas'. The 'Koshas' are:

1) The Anamaya Kosha Level Practices: These are at the physical level and include cleansing routines or 'kriyas', loosening exercises and yoga asanas

2) The Pranamaya Kosha Level Practices: These are practices at the vital energy level through practice of proper breathing and pranayama. These practices enable awareness and control of "Prana' or life force and to remove imbalances caused by Prana abnormalities.

3) The Manomaya Level Kosha Practices: These are practices at the mind level. The techniques used here are meditation as described in the last three limbs of Ashtanga Yoga of Patanjali which are 'Dharana', 'Dhyana' and 'Samadhi'. Emotional balance is also made possible by Bhakti Yoga.

4) The Vijnanamaya Level Kosha Practices: These are practices at the intellectual level and include a basic understanding and realization that happiness is within each one of us and is like the causal 'Ananda' state. This 'inner Jnana' can clear the mind, relieves

all doubts and removes wrong habits, agitations, hence providing grounding and stability to the body and mind. This knowledge is contained in the Upanishads and helps remove obsessions, likes and dislikes that agitate the mind and finds the sources of happiness through this inner Jnana.

5) The Anandamaya Level Kosha Practices: These are practices at the bliss level and Karma Yoga helps to de-identify oneself from the ups and downs in situations. Bliss being our true nature, is becoming farfetched thanks to the present day lifestyle, goal oriented working environments and increasing problems of stress. Karma Yoga helps in psychological corrections by enabling action with bliss and relaxation.

Setup and Practice

To set up your yoga practice you will need

- ➢ A clean and silent place

- ➢ A yoga mat

- ➢ A pair or two of lightweight yoga blocks

- ➢ A yoga strap

- ➢ A hand towel

- ➢ A bottle of warm water

- ➢ Some pillows and cushions

- ➢ Pens and notebooks

YOGA ROUTINE

Our body is constituted of 5 elements: water, air, fire, water and space. For our body to be healthy, these elements have to be in balance. Yoga enables balance with its many techniques and secrets. For this, a 75 minutes yoga practice must include the following practices as part of the normal routine:

- Prayer, yogic breath and om chanting 4 minutes

- Yog Agni Fire of Yoga and Head rotations or Brahma Mudra 2 minutes

- Warm up exercises 5 minutes

- Moving with your breath : Sun salutation 3 rounds

Or Yogic jogging + mukh dhauti 4 minutes

☐ Moving with your breath: The yoga asanas as planned   45 minutes

☐ Pranayama, Meditation and Omkara 15 minutes

- Yog Agni Fire is rubbing of palms together until they are warm and then placing them over the eyes

- Brahma Mudra is neck movements synchronized with deep breathing and 'Nada' or vibrational sounds

Suggested References: 'The heart of yoga' by TB Desikachar

'Asana Pranayama Mudra Bandha' by Swami Satyananda Saraswati

CHAPTER 2: YOGIC DIET

YOGIC DIET

A proper diet is a necessity for good health and emotional wellbeing and has an influence on our thoughts and spiritual progress. Ayurveda, a natural sister science of yoga, considers food as medicines. Ayurveda classifies food as well as people into three categories namely 'vata', 'pitta', and 'kapha'. Though everyone has the qualities of all three components, each person has a prominent, a less prominent and a least prominent presence. The imbalance of the components of a person is called a 'dosha'.

The three categories of food whose imbalance causes health imbalances or 'doshas' are

- Pitta or hot and oily; composed of fire and water; governs the digestive and metabolic system. Pitta foods are hot and/or oily.

- Vata or dry and light, composed of ether and air, governs movement. Vata foods are light and/or dry.

- Kapha or cold and moist, composed of earth and water, governs lubrication and structure. Kapha foods are cold and/or moist.

A yogic diet prescribes the necessary food for good health. The food required can be roughly identified with the help of the following table and is also dependent on the climate and season of the year.

	Pitta Food	Vata Food	Kapha Food
Pitta Dosha (concerning digestion and metabolism)	No	Moderate	Yes
Vata Dosha (concerning movement)	Yes	No	Moderate
Kapha Dosha (concerning lubrication and structure)	Moderate	Yes	No

Food is traditionally classified into three categories according to the influence they have on our mind and body.

- Sattvic food is pure and harmonious to our wellbeing. They help spiritual aspirants maintain a still and quiet mind. Examples are dairy products, fruits and vegetables, cereals and lentils. Other aspects of sattvic food include eating to live and not living to eat, eating quietly without talking and with awareness and at a moderate rate. Habits like moderate pace and mindfulness in eating can also be of a sattvic nature. Food can be satvik if the stomach is only half filled with food, a quarter with water and a quarter empty after eating a meal.
- Rajasic food influences the activity and passion levels and can also result in an overactive mind. Rajasic food includes meat, fish, hot and spicy food such as chillies, onions and garlic. A little rajasic food (e.g. hot spices that can help in digestion), can be satvik in nature.
- Tamasic food results in sluggishness and can lead to slowness, apathy and even a torpid state of mind that can hamper clear thinking. Other effects include dullness in mind and body, negative moods and inertia. These foods are decayed, stale and fermented food such as alcohol, drugs, tobacco, ill cooked food, overripe vegetables, overeating is also tamasic.

Cooking the food alters the state of the food and can make the food as satvik, rajasic or tamasic. This is done by combination with other foods and spices. For example; some foods like honey which is satvik when eaten as it is, becomes tamasic if it is cooked.

Non vegetarian foods are not allowed according to the recommendation of the hatha yoga pradipika, because the fear of death would have permeated each and every cell of the animal when it was slaughtered and when eaten have an adverse effect. The hatha yoga pradipika recommends lacto vegetarian food that excludes eggs, meat and fish. Even modern research has found that people on a vegetarian diet are healthier than people on a non - vegetarian diet. A better quality of proteins than that of meat can be obtained from nuts, dairy products, lentils and legumes.

Indicated:

- A general sattvic diet, a balanced attitude
- Eating at regular timings
- Do not speak while eating and observing silence
- A two hour gap between food and exercise
- At least a three hour gap between dinner and sleep

YOGIC LIFESTYLE

A yogic lifestyle includes a general sattvic diet and a balanced lifestyle. A balanced lifestyle includes a balanced attitude, having suitable recreational activities and a stable environment. A balanced lifestyle also includes having regular sleep, regular and healthy exercise that brings emotional stability.

An individual can keep fit by imbibing simple routine habits like waking up early and going to bed early. Simple good routines can bring radical changes to the body, mind and consciousness:

'Pratidinam kartavya charyaa dinacharya' which means that those activities that we perform regularly as a habit are called Dinacharyaa. These habits include:

- ➢ Personal conduct
- ➢ Social conduct
- ➢ Diet and fasting
- ➢ Maun

PERSONAL CONDUCT

1. Waking up early during BRAHMA MUHURTA (4 - 6 AM). The Panchamahabhutas which are the five elements: earth, water, air, fire and ether are in a pure state at this time and it is the most pure and fresh time of the day and keeps one fresh all through the day.

    Contraindications: It is not necessary if on waking up the food is still feeling like it is undigested. This practice may not suit the very young or old people, parents with small children and people suffering from diseases.

2. Natural urges: One should have a proper urge to defecate naturally and the best time for elimination is in the morning. The previous day's diet naturally has an effect on the next day's natural urges. Some good practices in exercise and diet can help in this respect.

3. Regular exercise or yoga is essential to remove stagnation in the body and to improve strength and endurance and help maintain the normal functioning of the body.

4. Abhangya is self-massage with oil. It helps us keep strong and prevents us from aging. Massaging the scalp, forehead, temples, hand and feet for 5 minutes a day is sufficient.

5. Brushing the teeth regularly with a good toothpaste and with neem sticks which have antibacterial properties, should be done. Regular rinsing of the mouth with cold water during summers and warm water during winters and cleaning of the tongue is to be done for fresh breath.

6. Ears can be cleaned daily by kriya, nose by jala neti and eyes by kriya.

7. Daily bathing is cleansing and refreshing and should not be done immediately after a meal. Having a bath with cold water has also been a good practice.

8. Eating meals breakfast, lunch and dinner; should be at regular timings after offering salutations to God and maintaining a calm and pleasant state of mind throughout the mealtimes. Food should be what you are accustomed to and the meals should be enriched with all six rasas or tastes namely sweet, astringent, bitter, sour, hot and salty. Food should be easily digestible and a part of the stomach to be left empty.
Contraindications: stale food or eating food while depressed and sleeping immediately after food, strenuous activities after food.

9. Remembering God or having good thoughts before sleeping. Though all directions are good, the head should preferably be facing East or South directions.

SOCIAL CONDUCT

1. Good interpersonal relations by respecting the elders, teachers and forefathers and so on
2. Helping and empathetic attitude towards the elderly, the ailing and the weak, physically challenged.
3. Sharing joy and achievements with well wishers
4. Not to give authority to unknown persons
5. Not to rely on anyone completely
6. Not to disclose other people's secrets in public
7. Speaking with the context of truth and in ones turn

8. Avoid people who are ill mannered or have evil thoughts
9. Not doing the following - lying, anger, extreme grief, extreme greed, jealousy, gossiping, ill - commenting, sins, unhealthy criticism, enmity towards others

DIET AND FASTING

Diet therapy is with food taken in its natural form. Example - fresh seasonal fruits and vegetables, green leafy vegetables and sprouts. To improve health and to purify and strengthen the body against diseases, food should be 20% acidic and 80% alkaline based. 'Therapy' diets considers food as medicines and can be classified into three forms:

1. Eliminative diet : These are detoxing and cleansing and include lemon juice and other citric juices, tender coconut water, vegetable soups, buttermilk, green leafy based juices and so on
2. Soothing diet: These are based on the whole and natural form of fruits, salads, boiled and steamed vegetables, vegetable chutneys and pastes
3. Constructive diet: These include carbohydrates and protein like whole wheat flour, unpolished rice with some curd, pulses and sprouts

Fasting techniques depend on the nature of the requirement; whether it is done to maintain health or to cure a disease. Fasting helps to burn up and excrete huge amounts of accumulated wastes in the body. Fasting should be done with natural foods by choosing to take only water or some fruit juices or some raw vegetable juices. At the end of fasting, food should be consumed in moderation and chewed slowly before transitioning into a normal diet. Calorie fasting and intermittent fasting are helpful in combating stress and to enhance immunity.

MAUN

Maun is a communication tool to communicate with the atma or self. Maun is the cessation of speaking by mouth and the mind. Maun has significant benefits for the Yoga aspirants and practice can be daily for 4 hours.

'Maun enables spiritual listening to the earth, its oceans, its underworld and also to the universe. By this type of listening, sins are washed away, pains are reduced, bliss and Shakti arise where even death cannot touch the practitioner and the secrets of yoga and its technology are learned.' The mind becomes calmer and is able to assimilate the knowledge of the scriptures more easily and life becomes much less stressful and more productive.

REFERENCES: Yoga and Naturopathy for Holistic Health by Department of Ayurveda, Government of India

CHAPTER 3: ASANAS AND THE TEACHING METHODOLOGY

ASANAS PRANAYAMAS and meditation are some techniques in yoga that have to be done on an empty stomach. It is recommended that there be a 3 hour gap after meals and before practicing asanas. When practicing asanas, put your whole concentration into it. The movement within and between asana is in perfect synchrony with the breathing. Generally inhalations are followed by extensions and exhalations are followed by contraction of the belly. Focus within yourself and your breathing and do not dwell in the past or ponder over the future.

About asanas
Stirram - to find the pose and be still
Sukham - to experience happiness and contentment

Asana is the first practice in hatha yoga but has the third place in Ashtanga yoga. There are many benefits of yoga asanas including

- Stable and strong body

- Health and fitness of mind, body and emotions

- Weight management

- Relationship improvement

- Relieves stress tension and anxiety

- Inner peace pleasure and bliss

- Increased immune power

- Flexible body

- Relieves diseases

- Balanced life

General Classification of Asanas

- Warm up exercises or Sukshma Vyayama

- Meditation asanas - Sukhasana, siddhasana

- Standing asanas

- Sitting asanas

- Lying asanas: Spine and Prone positions

- Joint Movement Exercises

- Twisting asanas

- Inversion asanas

- Balancing asanas - maybe on one hand, one leg, on the hip or on the arms

- Forward bending pose

- Backward bending pose - also in the sitting , standing and lying down positions

- Padmasana group asanas

- Ek pad group asanas

- Vinyasa, Surya Namaskars and Chandra Namaskars

You can mix all these asanas and make the class

Asana Variations

- Start the class with standard opening poses and simple postures
- In the asana poses, one posture can have different modifications
- These modifications are made according to the the objective of the class and requirement and body type of the students
- Divide the poses into normal , intermediate and advanced practice
- Demonstrate the pose or show the posture on the screen or give the demonstration) and time for practice

Posture:
- When you hold a movement it becomes a posture
- Posture means stability - This is asana and this is where you inhale and exhale
- You have to also focus on pranayama practice

STANDING POSES

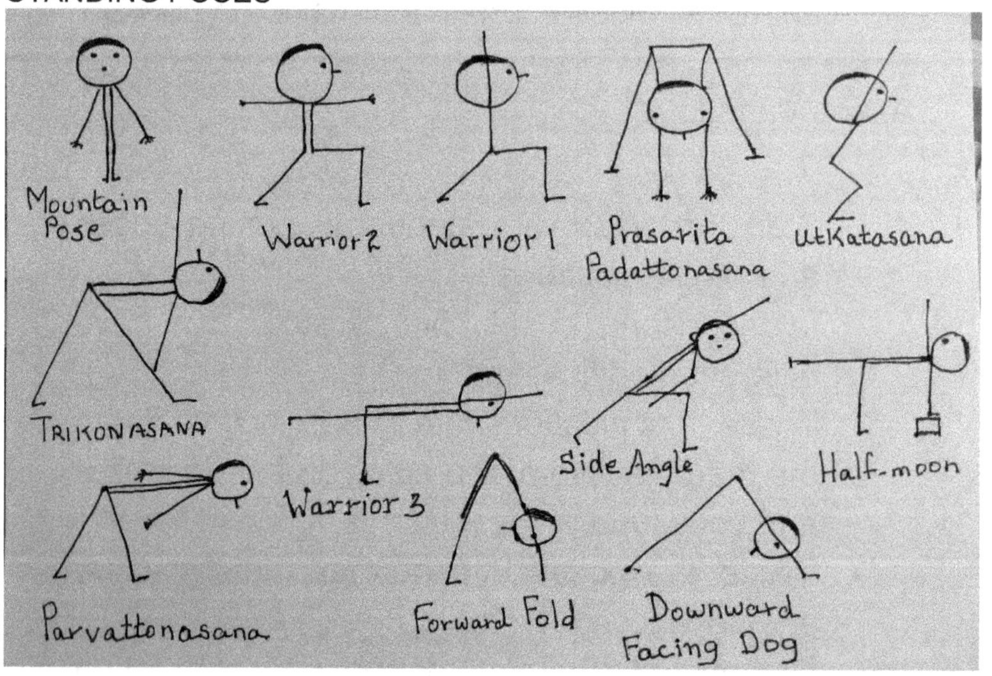

SITTING POSES

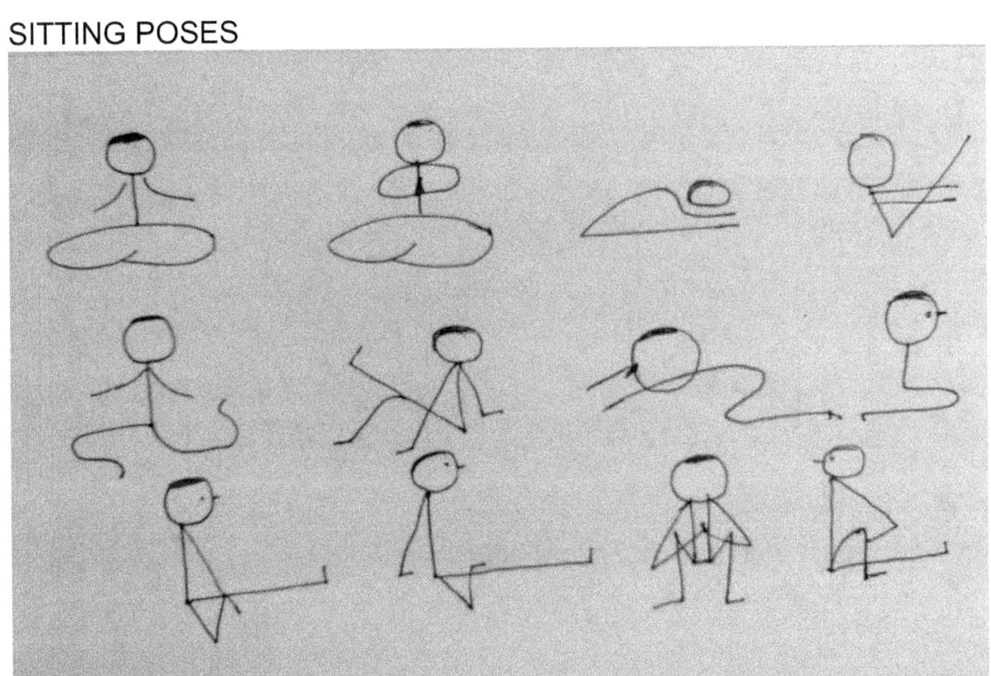

TWISTING POSES

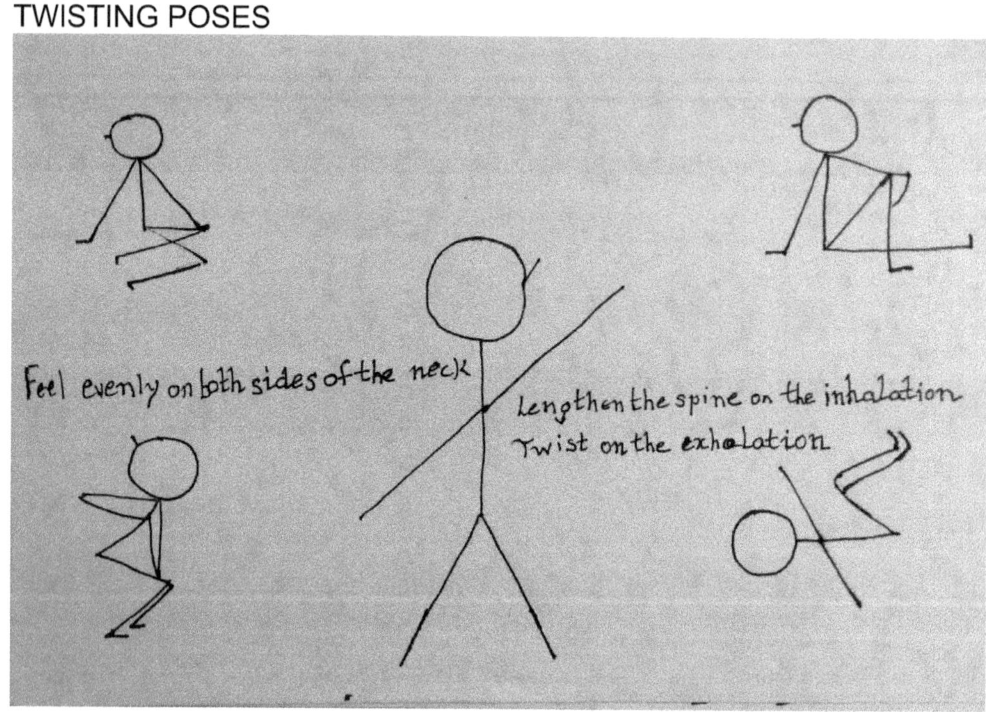

FORWARD BENDING POSES

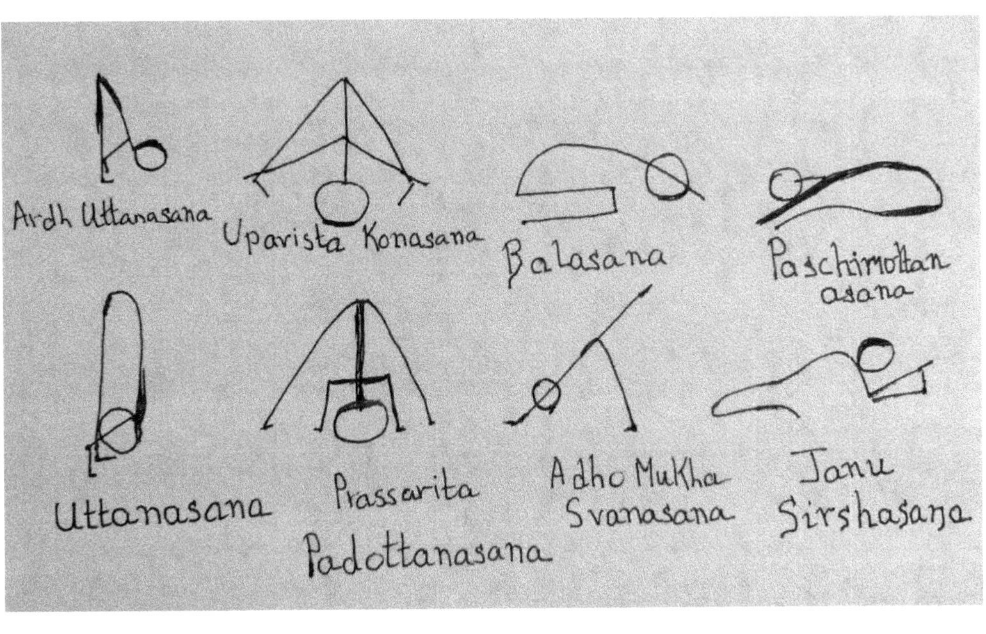

ARM BALANCES POSES

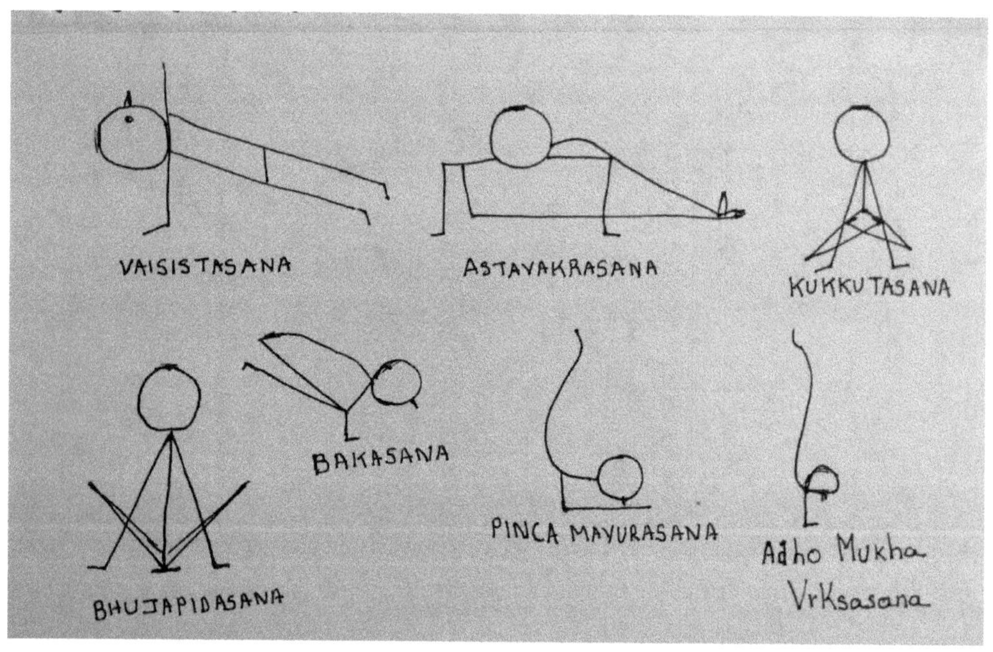

CORE ASANA POSES

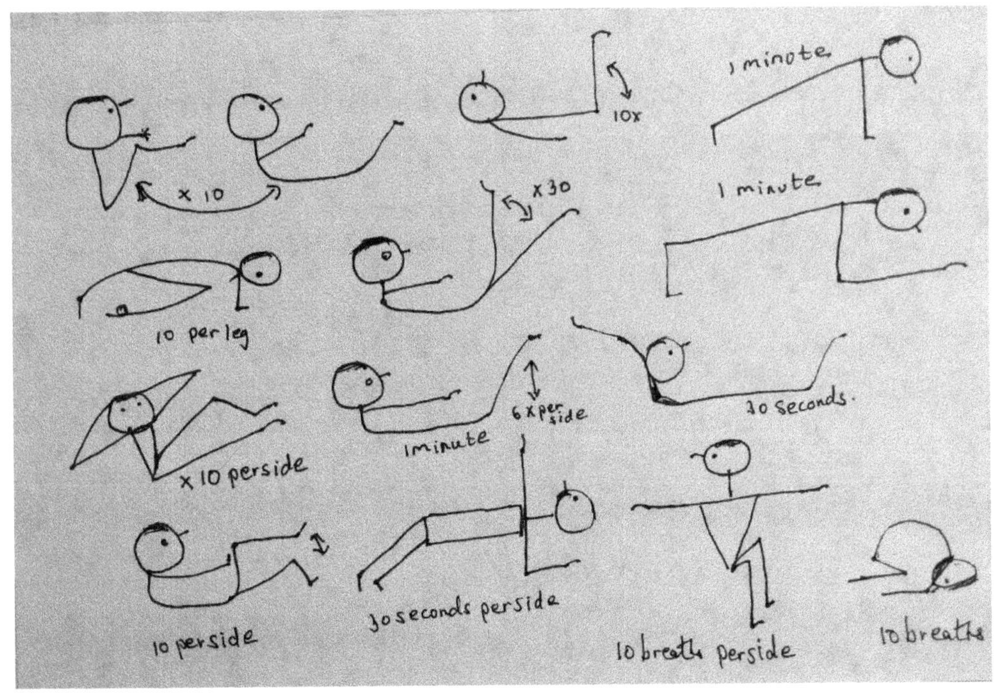

BACKBEND POSES

Ekpada RajaKapotasana (1)

Raja Kapotasana

Urdva Dhanurasana .

Ekpada Ustrasana

Kapotasana

Ekpada RajaKapotasana (2)

Laghu Vajrasana

Dhanurasana

Bhujangasana

INVERSION POSES

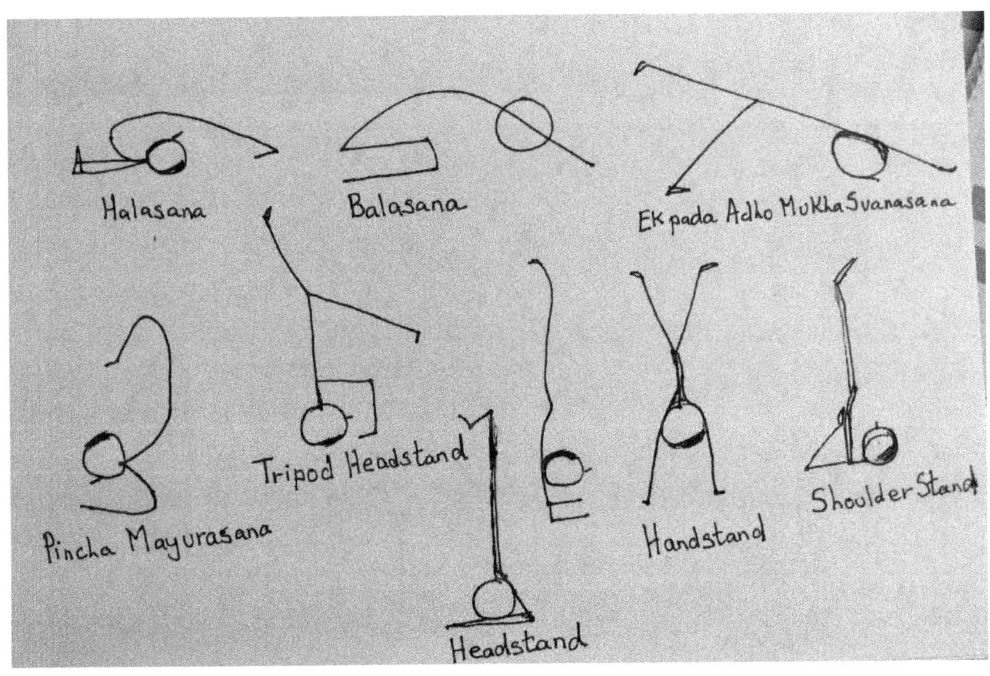

BALANCING POSES

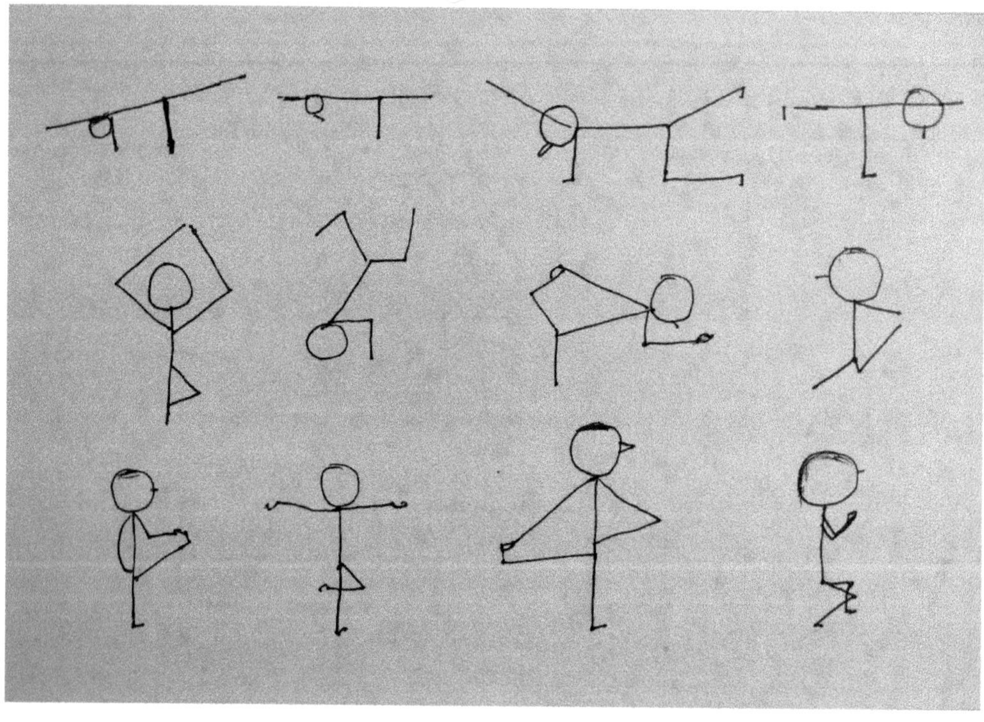

RESTORATIVE POSES

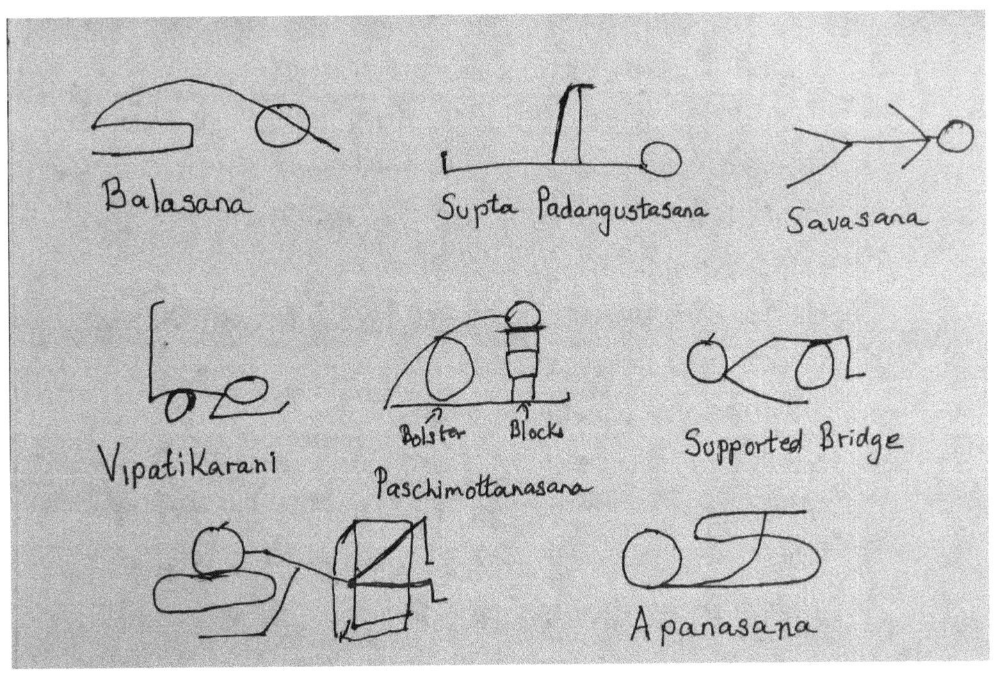

Asana Alignment in Sun Salutation

Inhale: Tadasana with namaste mudra
- Padam bandha
- Inhale hands up exhale bend back - spine lifting
- If the leg is between arms then neck will be lengthening
- Flexibility according to person
- Palms together or Fingerlock is all ok

Exhale Uttanasana - Front Forward Fold
- Standing with feet together, fold or bend forward
- Hold toes or ankles or the calf's or try and keep your palms on the mat
- Bend the upper body at the hips and keep your head downwards
- Uttanasana Modifications:
  Look up - look sideways - look down
  Movement - down and up - twist right and left
  - go front go back - leg sideways bend knees -
  .these movements are good to reduce weight

Inhale - Ashwa Sanchalanasana - Low Lunge
- Put leg back and look to the front
- Knee and ankle should be aligned
- If arms are short you can arch the fingertips - you can use the block
- Elbow position - elbows should be facing each other
- Knee in between the arms - no need to touch legs

- In Salutations the arm position should remain the same
- Knees can be up or down

Exhale and Inhale - Phalakasana - Plank Pose
- Put the other leg back which means that both legs are taken back
- Keeping a gap between the arms; being the shoulder and the wrist aligned with each other (same as the cat posture or any arm using pose)
- Shoulder away from the ears
- The toes are aligned with heels
- Knees- legs should be straight
- Once you come in the pose you should tuck the belly in
- The spine should be straight
- Sinking shoulder can cause a problem for the wrist and elbow
  (Plank modifications:
  Forearm Plank: For forearm plank everything remains the same - only drop elbows
  Side Plank - In the side plank you arch sideways with one arm up, the elbows should be facing in - the wrist elbow and shoulder should be aligned
  In the side plank you can bend your knee, move your leg up and down or move your leg front and back - you can touch your toe. Good idea for yoga for weight loss series)

Exhale: Eight Limbed Pose - Ashtanga Namaskar
- To touch the Mother Earth
- Position of the arms - the elbows closer to the body

- The fingertips and the shoulders should be aligned
- Shoulders should be away from the ears
- Lower body part - curl the toes inside and lift the hips up- bring the awareness on the tailbone
- Chin should be towards the chest

Correlating plank and ashtanga namaskar:
In plank the elbow should be facing inside
But when going to ashtanga namaskar or chaturanga, the elbows are facing inside as they are bending, Keeping the shoulder and wrist aligned and the shoulders away from the ears require a lot of strength
So do little at a time for practice
Otherwise - you can drop knees and hold plank position to transition to chaturanga or ashtanga namaskar and then you can practice this transition with lifting knees
Otherwise the transition can be made by lying down with the chest and just lifting the hip up a little
You can find your own way

Inhale:

Urdhva Mukha Svanasana - Upward dog (modern style)
- Lift your hip up and push chest in between arms and shoulders away from the ears push shoulder back so that you can use the whole spine
- Heels aligned feet can be together or apart
- You can tuck your toes until you transition to he next pose which is downward facing dog

Or

Cobra pose or bhujangasana (traditional style)
- Lift up your head and chest keeping elbows bending. Push your chest in between your arms and shoulders away from your ears and push your shoulders back so that you can use the whole spine
- You can tuck your toes until you transition to he next pose which is downward facing dog

Exhale: Adho Mukho Svanasana - Downward Facing Dog
- From ashtanga namaskar, press your palms and feet back and raise your hips up and back for downward facing dog on the palms and feet
- Spread your fingers wide on the mat and press through all of your fingers and the base of your palms
- Inhale and press your shoulders down, exhale and push your hip out and back
- For longer time in downward facing dog, find your bandhas : mula bandha, uddiyana bandha and jalandhara bandha

Inhale: Ashwa Sanchalana - Low Lunge
- From downward facing dog put leg forward
- Knees can be up or down

Exhale: Uttanasana
- Both feet together front forward fold

Inhale - Tadasana

- Both hands up, hands straight and legs straight
- Bend back a little

Homework

Work hard - make a picture in each of these modifications and keep them on a file

CHAPTER 5: PRANAYAMA

Breathing is necessary in daily life and in yoga. The technique of breathing is called as pranayama. Pranayama is generally defined as breath control
- Pranayama = Prana + Yama
- Pranayama has 2 roots - pran-im

Prana = vital energy or life force, it is a force which exists in all things and yama means to gain control Although closely related to the air we breathe, prana is more subtle than air or oxygen, therefore Pranayama should not be considered a mere breathing exercise. It is aimed at introducing extra oxygen into the lungs and also elevates the prana shakti or the life shakti's.

Pranayama utilizes breathing techniques to influence the flow of prana into the nadi's or energy channels of our body

In the Pranayama practice, there are 4 aspects of breathing which are utilized

1. Purak or inhalation
2. Rechaka or exhalation
3. Antarya kumbhaka - breath retention after inhalation
4. Bahya kumbhaka - breath retention after exhalation

The most important part of Pranayama is kumbhaka or breath retention. To perform kumbhaka successfully, there must be a gradual development of control over the functions of respiration. Therefore in the practice of Pranayama, more emphasis is given to inhalation and exhalation at the beginning and in order to strengthen the lungs and balance the nervous and pranic systems in preparation for the practice of kumbhaka. These practices influence the flow of prana in the nadis, purifying, regulating and activating them.

Best practices for pranayama:
- Always breathe through the nose not from the mouth unless specifically {mukha dhauti or murcha pranayama)
- During pranayama the nose should be cleaned
- You can clean the nose regularly by jala neti

THE TYPES AND THE MAIN TECHNIQUES OF BREATHING

1. Natural Breathing - Natural breathing happens when we sleep, eat, walk, we are not aware so it's natural
2. Abdominal Breathing
- All the air into stomach

3. Chest breathing
- Take all the air into the lungs to give more oxygen to the lungs

4. Yogic breathing- combines all the three techniques
   - Natural breathing
   - Abdominal breathing
   - Thoracic (chest) breathing

Yogic Breathing is used to maximize inhalation and exhalation. Its purpose is to gain control of the breath, correct poor breathing habits and create oxygen. It may be practiced at any time and it is useful in situations of high stress or anger for calming the nerves.

How to do yogic Breathing
- Sit in any meditative posture or lying down in savasana and relax the whole body. Inhale slowly and deeply allowing the abdomen to expand fully
- Try to breathe so slowly, the sound should be little no sound
- When doing this process feel the air reaching to the bottom of the abdomen and lungs - At the end of abdominal expansion, start to expand the chest outwards and upwards - When the ribs are fully expanded, inhale little more until expansion is felt in the upper portion of the lungs and over the base of the neck
- When doing this process, the shoulders and the collar bone should also move up slightly - Feel a little bit tension in the neck area
- The rest of the body should be relaxed
- Feel the air in the lungs
- This completes one inhalation
- The whole process will be continuous
- After that start to exhale
- First relax the lower neck and upper chest
- Then allow the chest to contract downward and inwards
- Allow the diaphragm to push upward and towards the chest
- Without straining try to empty the lungs as much as possible by pulling the abdomen as near as possible to the spine
- At the end of exhalation, hold the breath for a

few seconds
- This is a complete round of yogic breathing

At first the beginning performs 5 -10 rounds and slowly increases it to 10 minutes daily (You should have awareness of the movement of the breath)

5. Balancing pranayama involve rechaka, kumbhaka and puraka and the ida and pingala nadis

    Suryabedhan - Surya is sun and bedhan means revealing the secret. It is a stimulating practice or activation of fire in our body system and it stimulates pingala nadi on the right nostril. When pingala nadi is active, alertness and vitality are heightened. Benefits of Surya Bhedana: there are many physical benefits of this pranayama which includes and creates physical energy and mental alertness. It also increases heat in the body and it's also helpful for the awakening of prana. Therapeutic benefits: relief from depression and reduction of overweight, oversleeping, cold cough and gastric ailments. Performing suryabhedana continuously is good for the purification of the skull and for eliminating abdominal disease

    Technique

    Sit in sukhasana or any comfortable easy pose with a still body, nasika mudra, slowly inhale and exhale from the right side by closing the left nostril. We can add the Kumbhak also

Perform Kumbhak until the air diffuses into the roots of the spine and to the tips of the nails of the feet and hands.

You can also exhale; rechak. from the left nostril

Chandrabedhan

In Sanskrit Chandra means moon and bedhan means revealing the secret of the moon. The complementary practice of Suryabhedana is Chandrabedhana.

Concentrate the breath into the left nostril or ida nadi which is the channel responsible for more calm and receptive energy. It can also be performed by closing the right nostril and inhaling and exhaling from the left side

Benefits: can be used to relax our body and mind and it's also relief from anxiety, insomnia and for cooling the body and relax and peace of mind

Therapeutic benefits

It helps migraine allergies skin problems

Technique

Sit in any comfortable pose with a straight back, relax the whole body and mind and keep the eyes closed.

Inhale exhale from left

Inhale from left and exhale from right

Anulom Vilom and **nadi shodhana** - Nadi shodhana and anulom vilom alternate breathing.

Nadis are invisible energy channels like the energy nerves in our body. Shodan means purification, Nadi shodhana means a pranayama which purifies our nadis. As per yogic science we have 72000 nadis. In the human body some are called purush. The structure and operation of the human body is like a large city, 72000 streets which we need to keep clean. This can be done easier with the nadi shodhana pranayama. Some yogis also call this pranayama as anulom vilom. Anulom means straight and vilom means reverse. In this technique the duration of inhalation and exhalation is controlled. The purpose of the pranayama is to clean and purify and cleanse the nadis

Technique

Sit in sukhasana or padmasana with head, neck and spine in a straight line and keep the left hand in chi or gyan mudra on the left knee. Make nasika mudra with your right hand and close your eyes. Begin inhaling from the left nostril and retain the breath inside, then close the left nostril and open the right nostril. Slowly exhale from the right nostril and then inhale through the right nostril and retain and then exhale through the left nostril. The whole procedure we should do with awareness.

There are several ways to perform alternate nostril breathing. Each involving unique rhythm of inhaling purak, internal retention or antar kumbhaka and exhaling, retaining exhalation or bhayaya kumbhaka

Ratio and timing: After a few days of practice, if there are no difficulties, you can increase the length of inhalation and exhalation in your count

Do not force the breath and after holding breath. Practice to the best of your abilities

Benefits

This breathing technique balances the nervous system and the energetic channels. It brings balance to the mind. When the flow of prana is equal in both ida and pingala nadi, it can begin to enter sushumna nadi. Sushumna nadi is the central channel which allows kundalini energy to rise. All the chakras lie within the sushumna nadi.

Ratio and timing: The maintenance of a strict ratio during inhalation, kumbhaka and exhalation is important. The ratio will change as the ability to hold the breath for longer periods of time changes. So, master the ratio of 1:1:1; after that increase the ratio to 1:1:2. For example inhale for a count of 5 then perform internal Kumbhak for a count of 5 and then exhale for a count of 10. After some weeks of practice when this ratio has been mastered, increase the ratio to 1:2:2. After mastering the ratio of 1:2:2, increase the count by adding 1 unit to the inhalation, 2 units to the retention and 2 units to the exhalation.

6. Cleansing pranayama
   - Bhastrika
   - Kapalbhati

7. Pranic energy locking pranayama
   - Ujjayi pranayama
   - Murcha
   - Pavani

8. Soothing pranayama

- Bhramari

9. Cooling pranayama
    - Sheetali
    - Sheetkari

CHAPTER 6: MUDRAS, MANTRAS AND BANDHAS

Mudra is a Sanskrit word and it is a sign in yoga and has many meanings like

- Pose
- Money
- Seal
- Impression

Mudras are used for many purposes for channeling the subtle energies and powers. Mudras have the capacity to lessen our weakness and bring about complete health. Mudras may involve the whole body in a combination of asana pranayama bandha or it may be a simple hand position.

Outline of the palms:

Positioning the fingers and the thumb in a particular manner enables the flow of energy between them in a manner that enhances specific brain and body functions

- Thumb signifies agni and fire

- Index signifies air; vayu and regulates and represents the air in the body

- Middle finger signifies akash space; regulates the akash tatwa

- Ring finger signifies prithvi earth

- Little finger signifies jal, water

1. Hasta (hand) mudras:

Hasta mudras redirect the prana being emitted by the hand back into the body
Mudras which join the thumb and index fingers engage the motor functions. The main types of hasta mudras are jnana mudra and chin mudra.

Janan mudra - Hold the index finger so that they touch the inside root of the thumb and straighten the other fingers of each hand so that they are relaxed and slightly apart. Place the hands on to the knees with palms facing down and relax your hands and arms. Janan mudra is a gesture of knowledge

Chin mudra: Chin mudra is performed in the same way as Janan mudra except that the palms of both hands face upwards. With the back of the hands resting on the knees. Relax the hand and arms
Benefits of janan and chi mudra are simple but important physio natural fingerlock which make meditation asanas more powerful. The palms and fingers of the hands have many nerve roots and which constantly emit energy. Hasta mudras increase memory power and sharpness of the brain. Chin mudra is a gesture of consciousness. It also increases the learning capacity. It increases the smooth flow of blood supply in the brain. When the palms face upward In the chin mudra, the chest area is opened up. So the practitioner may experience this as a sense of lightness
Time duration: normally there is no particular time duration. You can practice while standing, sitting or

while lying down whenever and wherever you have the time

2. **Yoni mudra**

This mudra signifies the attitude of the whole. As you make comfortable meditation posture with head and spine straight

Place the palms of the hands together with the fingers and the thumbs. Point the fingers downwards keeping the thumbs straight and pointing away from the body. Keep the back of the index fingers together. Turn the little, ring and middle fingers inwards so that the back of the fingers are touching.

Benefits: the interlocking of the fingers in this practice creates a connection of energies from the right hand to left hand and vice versa. It also balances the energies in the body. It also helps to balance the activities of the right and left hemispheres of the brain. Thus mudra makes the body and mind more stable in meditation. It develops greater concentration awareness and internal physical relaxation

3, **Varun mudra**

This mudra is of water

Method: The tip of the little finger touches the tip of thumb with other three fingers stretched out

Speciality: It balances the water content, it prevents all diseases which comes due to lack of water, it balances water content in the body and it prevents the pain of muscle shrinkage and gastroenteritis

Practice according to your time

4. Vayu mudra

Mudra of air

Method Keep the index finger on the base of the thumb and press with thumb while keeping the other three fingers straight with both hands

Speciality: it prevents all the diseases that occur due to the imbalance of air

Time duration: practice this mudra for 45 minutes. The severity of the disease is reduced in 12 - 24 hours

Practice for 2 months for good results

Benefits: it cures arthritis, gout and paralysis without any medicine

It corrects cervical spondylitis, paralysis to face and nerve pinching in the neck

It also corrects the disorder of gas in the stomach

5. Shunya mudra

Mudra of emptiness

Keep the middle finger at the root of the thumb and press it with thumb

Speciality: reduces dullness in the body

Time duration- 40 -60 minutes daily

Benefits:

It relieves early ache in 4-5 minutes

It also assists the weak and mentally challenged

6. Surya mudra

Mudra of sun

Bend the ring finger and press it with the thumb

It sharpens the center in the thyroid gland

Practice 2 times daily for 5-15 minutes

Benefits: it reduces cholesterol in the body and helps in reducing weight
It reduces anxiety
Corrects indigestion problems

7. Apana mudra

Mudra of digestion
Method: the tips of the middle finger and ring finger touch the tip of the thumb
It plays an important role in our health because it regulates the excretory system
Practice this mudra for 45 minutes
It regulates diabetes
It cures constipation and piles

8: Sanjeevani mudra

Mudra of heart
Method: the tips of the middle finger and ring finger touch the tip of the thumb while the index finger touch the base of the thumb
It benefits the heart and it's also helpful in heart attack
Practice many times as much as you can
The heart patient and blood pressure patient can practice for 15 minutes daily
It strengthens the heart and it helps with gastric troubles

9: Linga mudra

Mudra of heat
Method: interlock the fingers of both hands and keep the thumb of the left hand straight
And encircle it with the thumb and the index finger of the right hand

It generates heat in the body and it's more beneficial if you take milk ghee more water and fruit juice in addition to the practice of this mudra
You can practice anytime but don't practice a lot because it produces heat in the body
It can cause sweating even in winter if you practice it for longer time
It gives power to the lungs. It cures severe colds

10. Mahasir mudra

Mudra for relieving tension
Touch the tip of the thumb with the top of index and middle finger
Keep the ring finger into the fold of the thumb and stretch the little finger straight out
15 - 20 minutes
This mudra relieves all tension
Benefits
Relieves migraine, eyes from strain and back pain

11. Hakini mudra

Mudra for memory
Touch the tip of the corresponding fingers of each other's hand
Thus mudra improves memory power and it helps to improve concentration
Can practice it 15 minutes

12. Saman mudra

Mudra of digestion
The tips of all the fingers with tip of the thumb
Time duration: 20 minutes
It controls the digestive system

It digests food and nourishes the body
It also prevents and cures many problems related to the digestive system

13. Bhairav mudra

Shiva Shakti Mudra

One palm is placed on top of another. It can be practiced during meditation. When the right palm is placed over the left palm, it is known as bhairava mudra. When the left palm is placed over the right palm, it is known as bhairavi mudra.

This mudra has been known to bring harmony and balance to either sides or hemispheres of the brain. It provides strength and stability and a sort of meditation to the entire body and inner self

14. Hridaya mudra

Heart gesture

Place the hands on the knees, palms facing upwards. Bend the index finger and place it at the base of the thumb. One should be able to feel the pulse. Touch the thumb to the middle and ring fingers. Let the little finger be relaxed

Helps redirect prana towards the heart, balancing the blood pressure and helping with heart problems. Helps open the heart on a pranic and emotional level, releasing emotions and tensions.

Mantra

What is Mantra and why do we use this?
The word Manushya (man) is made of man (mind) and mind is like a wave which always moves and

flows with subconscious and conscious thoughts. Mind wants more and more which leads to back to back thoughts in life. Here, prayer is a way you can free yourself from the desire and you can enter into a zone where the mind is not completely filled with thoughts. And if prayers are done with a true heart, it will give you the experience of being connected with your true self. When the prayers start blossoming, then you will start feeling complete happiness and freedom from sadness. Here all the religions in the world have accepted one sound which is the sound of Om. Our science has also accepted that sound is also energy and Shakti. Before and after yoga and meditation practice, prayers help in getting rid of all pains and sorrows of life. So here we have the yogic method of prayers.

Method:
- Start in a sitting or standing way
- With closed eyes
- With namaste mudra or anjali mudra
- In the beginning, relax the entire body
- Just take 3-4 deep relaxing breaths connect with yourself
- Chant Om 3 times and rub your palms together for about 1 minute. This will invoke yoga agni in your palms
- Yoga agni provides energy to all the body systems from your palms, which helps to relieve the all the problems within the mind
- Cover your face with the palms bending the head forward
- This energy from your palms transforms your problems into pleasure and you start feeling the experience of happiness and lightness

- After that very slowly and gently come back and open your eyes
- You are ready for the other yoga practice
- Before starting other yoga practice close your eyes and Chant the prayer
- Chant om 3 times very clearly and deep with 50 percent time open your mouth and 50.percent time close your lips and with full awareness then chant the prayer
- Prayer helps in making the mind stable and concentrated and it will relieve you from sadness, sorrows and suffering

Om sahana bhavatu
Sahanau bhunaktu
Saha viryam karva vahi
Tejas vinaa
Vadhitamastu
Maa vidhwisha vahai
Om shanti shanti shanti

Meaning of this shloka or prayer

Oh lord protect all of us
And help us that we get the capacity to study and understand
We acquired the knowledge
With the acquisition of this knowledge
Let peace flow in us
And help us that we get brilliant
We don't hold any enmity against anyone
Om peace peace peace

After chanting

- Eyes closed rub your palms and place them over your eyes
- Feel the heat and take this energy
- Bend a little forward
- Slowly come back and gently open your eyes

At the end of all yoga practices close your eyes and chant this sloka after Om chanting

Om sarve bhavantu sukhinah
Sarve Santu nirravanamaya
Sarve Bhadrani pashyantu
Maa Kashif
Dukh bhag bhave
Om shanti shanti shanti

Oh lord may all be happy
May all be free from disease
May all have peace and happiness in their life
No one suffers from sorrows
Om peace peace peace

One more prayer

Om asato maa sadgamaya
Tomaso maa jyotir gamaya
Mrytonma
Amritam gamaya
Om shanti shanti shanti

Lead me from the unreal to the real
From darkness to light
From death to immortality

Try to chant 2 to 3 days
Try to pronounce it and learn it

Bandhas and Mahabandha

Bandhas

Bandhas affect the pranic bodies. The bandhas aim.to block the pranas in particular areas and redirect their flow into Sushumna nadi for the purpose of spiritual awakening. Bandhas may be practiced individually or incorporated with mudra and pranayama practice. When combined in this way they awaken the psychic faculties. The bandhas directly act on the three granthis - Brahma, Vishnu and Rudra granthi.

There are 4 bandhas
1. Jalandhara
2. Moola
3. Uddiyana
4. Maha bandha - a combination of first three

Jalandhara bandha: Throat lock
- First sit in padmasana Siddhasana with head and spine straight
- The knees should be in firm contact with the floor
- Those who cannot manage this, they can do Jalandhara bandha in the standing position
- Place the palms of the hands onto the knees
- Close the eyes and relax the whole body
- Inhale slowly and deeply and retain the breath inside

- While retaining the breath, bend the head forward and press the chin tightly against the chest
- Straighten the arms and lock them firmly into position pressing the knees down with the hands
- Hunch the shoulders upwards and forward
- This will ensure that the arms stay locked
- hold the breath
- Stay in the final position for as long as the breath can be held comfortably
- Relax the shoulders
- Then bend the arms and slowly release the lock
- Raise the head and then exhale
- After this repeat after the respiration system has returned to normal
- The practice may also.be performed with external breath retention

Duration

The Duration of the Jalandhara bandha should be as long as the practitioner is comfortably

Gradually increase this period by maintaining the count while retaining the breath

This practice may be repeated upto 5 times

Physical awareness: The physical awareness is at the throat pit

Spiritual awareness: The spiritual awareness is Vishuddhi or throat chakra

Benefit:

- Jalandhara bandha compresses the carotid sinuses which are located on the carotid arteries, the main arteries in the neck
- This sinus helps to regulate the circulatory and respiratory system
- Normally, a decrease of oxygen and increase of carbon dioxide in the body leads to an increased heart rate and heavier breathing
- By artificially exerting pressure on these sinuses this deficiency is prevented allowing for decreased heart rate and increased breath retention
- This practice produces mental relaxation relieving stress anxiety and anger

Moola Bandhas

Perineum Contraction

1st stage
- Sit in Siddhartha or any asana
- That pressure is applied to the genital region
- Close the eyes and relax the whole body
- Be aware of the natural breath for a short while
- Then focus the awareness on to the genital region
- Contract this region by pulling up all the muscles of the pelvic floor and relaxing them
- Continue to briefly contract and relax the genital as rhythmically and evenly as possible

2nd stage
- First adjust the tensions in the spine to help focus on the point of contraction

- Slowly contract the genital region and hold the contraction
- Continue to breathe normally do not hold the breath
- Be totally aware of the physical sensations
- Contract a little bit tighter but keep the rest of the body relaxed
- Contract only those muscles related to the mooladhara region
- In the beginning the anal and the urinary sphincters also contract
- But as greater awareness and control is developed, this will be minimized and eventually will cease
- Ultimately you will feel one point of movement against the heel
- Relax the muscles slowly and evenly
- Repeat 10 times with maximum contraction and total relaxation

Technique 2

- Moola bandha with internal breath retention
- Sit in a meditative asana so that the knees touch the floor - siddhasana
- Place the palms onto the knees
- Close the eyes and relax the whole body for a few minutes
- Inhale deeply and retain the breath inside and perform jalandhara bandha
- Maintain jalandhara bandha
- Perform moola bandha by slowly contracting the vaginal region and hold the contraction as tightly as possible
- Do not strain

- This is the final lock
- Hold it as long as the breath can comfortably be retained
- After that slowly release moola bandha and then raise the head to the upright position and exhale
- Practice upto 10 times
- Breathing: This practice can be done with the external breath retention

Physical Awareness
- While taking the final position and performing jalandhara bandha awareness should be directed to the breath
- In the final position, awareness should be fixed at the place of perineal contraction

Spiritual awareness: The spiritual awareness is on the breath and on the mooladhara chakra while contracting

Benefits
- Moola bandha have many physical mental and spiritual benefits
- It stimulates the pelvic nerves and it is also beneficial for ulcers, prostatitis
- This practice releases energy
- It is also effective in the treatment of psychosomatic and some degenerative illnesses
- Its effects spread throughout the body via brain and endocrine system, making it very beneficial.in cases of asthma and arthritis
- It also reduces depression

- Moola bandha is both a means to attain sexual control, brahmacharya and it enables sexual energy to be directed in the upward for spiritual developments or downward to enhance mental relations
- It also helps to relieve sexual frustrations or feelings of sexual guilt

Uddiyana Bandha: Abdominal Contraction

- Sit in Siddhartha or padmasana with spine erect and knees in contact with the floor
- You can also sit on a cushion or pillow
- Keep your hands on your knees then gently close your eyes then relax
- Breath in from the nostrils and exhale from your mouth with a whoosh
- Empty your lungs as much as possible and then whole the breath and then lean forward and press down on the knees with palms and straighten hands and raise the shoulders
- Do jalandhara bandha with chin towards the chest
- Contract the abdominal muscles inward and upward
- And then hold the abdominal lock and breath for as long as you can without straining
- After that then release the abdominal lock, bend the elbows and lower the shoulders raise the head and then slowly Inhale
- After that remain in this position until the respiration returns to normal and then begin to the next round
- Uddiyana bandha is performed only with external breath retention

Duration
Practice 3 rounds in the beginning
With practice you can increase it up to 10 rounds

Physical awareness: The physical awareness is on to the abdomen and synchronizing the breath in coordination with the abdomen

Spiritual awareness: The spiritual awareness is on the manipura chakra

Contraindications
Person who are suffering from stomach ulcer hernia, high blood pressure, heart disease and pregnant women should not practice this

Benefits
- Good for many abdominal and stomach ailments including constipation, indigestion and diabetes
- The digestive fire is stabilized
- The abdominal organs are all massaged and toned
- It also improves blood circulation and strengthens all the internal organs

Maha Bandha - Great lock

Sit In padmasana with your hands on the knees .Keep your spine straight and close your eyes and relax your whole body

- Breathe in deeply and slowly through your nose
- Exhale forcefully and completely from mouth
- Retain the breath outside

First jalandhara
Next uddiyana
Next moola bandha
In this order

- Hold all the bandhas and the breath until you can hold it comfortably

Then release
Moola
Uddiyana
Jalandhar
In that order

Inhale slowly
This is one round

Physical awareness: After performing the bandhas rotate the consciousness between the bandhas. Remain aware of each region for a few seconds and then move to the next.

Spiritual awareness: After performing the bandhas rotate the consciousness from the muladhara, manipura and the vishuddhi chakra. Remain aware of each chakra and then move to the next

Duration
Upton10 rounds

Benefits

Gives the benefit of all three bandhas and it affects the hormonal secretions and the pineal gland

SHATKARMA

Cleansing Techniques

Meaning

Hatha yoga describes 6 (shat) actions (karma) or Shatkarma. Shatkarma consists of 6 groups of purification practices. The shatkarmas are Neti, Dhauti, Nauli, Basti, Kapalbhatti and Trataka.

The aim of hatha yoga and therefore of the shatkarma is to create harmony between two major organic flows - ida in the left side and pingala in the right side.

The shatkarma is also used.to balance the three doshas

1. Kapha (water energy)
2. Pitta (fire energy)
3. Vatta (air energy)

According to both ayurveda and yoga, any imbalance within these energies can cause illnesses and can be balanced by shatkarma.

Shatkarma practices are used before pranayama and other yoga practices in order to purify the body by removing toxins.

Precautions: These should not only be read but also practiced under guidance of an experienced yoga practitioner

TECHNIQUES:

The six cleansing techniques are: Neti, Dhauti, Nauli, Basti, Kapalbhatti and Trataka

(1) Neti - A process of cleansing and purifying the nasal passages: Jala neti (water and salt) and sutra neti (rubber catheter).

(2) Dhauti - Dhauti is a series of internal cleansing techniques which are divided into four groups:
Mula Shodhana (rectal cleansing)
Sirsa dhauti (head cleansing) and danta dhauti (the cleaning of the teeth, tongue, ears and eyes)
Hrida dhauti (chest cleansing, is divided into danda dhauti, vaman dhauti, and vastra dhauti)
Antar Dhauti is the cleansing of the lower part of the stomach region or large intestine

The internal cleansing cleans the entire alimentary canal from mouth to anus and is divided into four practices:

- Shank Prakshalana - cleansing of intestine which are of two types: (Duggar(big) and Lagu(small)
- Agnisar kriya - Activating the digestive fire
- Kunjal kriya or vamal dhauti: cleansing the stomach with water
- Vastra Dhauti - for cleansing the intestine

(3) Nauli - a method of massaging and strengthening the abdominal organs

(4) Basti - A technique for washing and toning the large intestine

(5) Kapalbhati - A breathing technique for purifying and cleansing the frontal region of the brain

(6) Trataka - Blink less gazing. The practice of intense gazing at one point or object which develops the power of concentration

1. NETI

Jalal neti: Nasal cleansing with water

Preparation
- A special neti pot should be used for this
- The water should be boiled and cooled water or purified water and should be at body temperature mixed with salt (sea salt or rock salt and preferably not table salt)
- The proportion is 1 teaspoon salt for ½ liter of water
- We have to put the nozzle at the end the end of the mouth comfortably into the nostril so that the water will flow into one nostril and out from the other
- When you do neti, if you feel some burning sensation it means you do not have enough salt
- The addition of salt ensures the osmotic pressure of the water is equal to that of the body fluids
- If you add too much salt, then also you will have a burning sensation. The proportion of salt should be normal

Procedure
- Fill the neti pot with prepared water. Get ready while standing (you can stand and keep your hands on your thighs) or in a squatting position
- Then close the eyes and relax the whole body

- And then keep the head slightly on one side
- During the practice, whenever you breathe you have to breathe from the mouth
- You have to put the nozzle into the nostril and tilt the head in the opposite direction
- And after some time, the water will come from the other side
- After half the water is over, center the head
- If you have any mucus then remove it. You can have a towel also
- Then tilt the head the other side
- Repeat the same process
- You can do this 2- 3 times
- After completing this process the nostrils should be dried. To do this, stand erect, inhale through both the nostrils, and then close one nostril and breathe out repeatedly with the other. This is called as single nostril kapalbhati
- Then you can do kapalbhati with both the nostrils
- You and keep 4-5 neti pots if required for the full practice
- This practice should be done for 5 -10 minutes
- This practice should be done once daily in a week or on alternate days. It should not be done everyday

Physical Awareness
- Neti is related to breathing through the mouth
- Neti helps in relaxation of the body and breath
- The nozzle should be on and within the nostril
- The physical awareness is on the ajna chakra

- Ideally neti should be practiced in the morning before asana and pranayama

Precautions:
- Water should not be too hot or too cold
- Water should pass through the nose
- If any water enters through the mouth it means that the position of the head should be adjusted
- Make sure that the nose is properly dried after the practice otherwise the nose will feel irritated and manifest the symptoms a cold
- Do not blow the nose too hard as the remaining water can come through the ears

Contraindications:
- Those persons suffering from chronic bleeding in the nose should not do jala neti
- Those who have blockages or structural blockages shouldn't do

Benefits
- Jala neti removes mucus and pollution from the nasal passages and sinuses allowing air to flow without obstruction
- It helps to relieve allergies cold and sinus
- It relieves muscular tension of the face
- It has a cooling and soothing influence on the brain
- It is beneficial in the treatment of migraine
- It alleviates anxiety, anger, depression and dark circles
- It also improves the eyesight and helps heal hearing problem

Sutra Neti

Nasal cleansing with thread

Preparation

- This practice involves passing a length of cotton thread on rubber catheter through the nose
- The width is 4MMS and the length is 36-45 cm
- It is lubricated with butter, oil, ghee so that it can go easily into the nasal passages
- You can put the oil into the nose also

Technique:

- Take any comfortable position, standing or sitting and first relax the whole body
- Tilt the head slightly back
- Whichever nostril is more open you can put the sutra neti
- Hold the neti string, put it in the nose and tilt in downward
- Initially there may be some itching
- When the thread reaches through the back of the throat then insert the index finger or middle finger and thumb and take it out of the mouth
- Then you have to pull both ways with your hands
- After completing you can take it out from the mouth

Breathing

- Breath should come from the mouth

Duration

- It takes 5 minutes
- For beginners it may take time to learn the technique

Physical Awareness
  - Relaxing the body
  - Moving the sutra neti or catheter or thread

Spiritual Awareness
  - Ajana Chakra

Precautions
  - Do not use force under any circumstances, as the anterior of the nose is delicate and any undue force can cause damage to the nose
  - You can clean the catheter after the practice and reuse it
  - It is best not to try sutra neti until we do jala neti

Contraindications
  - Persons suffering from chronic bleeding from the nose should not do
  - Anyone suffering from nasal ulcers should take advice from the teacher or doctor before practicing sutra neti

Benefits
  - Normally the benefits are the same as jala neti. And it helps maintain the nasal hygiene by removing the dirt and bacteria trapped along with the mucous in the nostril

- Sinus , migraine and headache problems can be reduced with the sutra neti

2. DHAUTI

Purification is of two kinds:
- Antar Dhauti (internal cleaning)
- Bahar Dhauti (external cleaning)

Antar Dhauti can be made in the following ways.
Vastra Dhauti

Take a fine piece of muslin cloth, 3 inches wide and 15 feet long. The borders should be stitched well and no pieces of loose thread should be hanging from its sides. Wash it with soap before use and make it clean. Dip it in tepid water. Squeeze out the water and swallow one end of it little by little. On the first day, swallow only one foot. Keep it there for a few seconds and then take it out very slowly. On the next day swallow a little more and keep it for a few minutes and then take it out slowly. Thus little by little you can swallow the whole length, retain it for about 5 minutes and then take it out. Do not be hasty. Do not injure your throat by rough handling. When the Kriya is over, drink a cup of milk. This is a sort of lubrication for the throat. This exercise should be done when your stomach is empty. Morning time is good. You do not need to practice this every day. Once in four days or once in a week is sufficient. This exercise cannot at all do any harm if gradually practiced. Everyone will feel a little vomiting sensation on the first 2 or 3 attempts. As soon as the Kriya is over, wash the cloth with soap and keep it always clean. This is an excellent exercise for those who are of a flabby and phlegmatic constitution.

Benefits:

Gradual steady practice cures gulma, gastritis, dyspepsia, diseases of the stomach and spleen, disorders of phlegm and bile. This exercise is also known as Vastra Dhauti. This is one variety of Antar Dhauti.

Shankh Prakshalan Kriya: See the section 'Shankh Prakshalan' for more information. There are some people who can drink plenty of water and pass it through the anus immediately. It is called "Varisara Dhauti". This is an effective method. This exercise is also known as 'Shankh Prakshalan Kriya'. This is not possible for the vast majority of people. Nauli and Uddiyana Bandha should be combined for performing this exercise. Even the smoke of a cigarette can be passed out through the anus. This is also a kind of purification exercise.

Internal cleaning can be made also by swallowing air. Fill up the stomach with plenty of air. It is done by hiccough. Just as you swallow food little by little, so also you can swallow air and fill up the stomach and intestines. You will have to learn this from the person who can do this Kriya. When you contract the abdominal muscles, the air will pass away through the anus as Apana Vayu. Those who can fill up their stomach with air can float on water just like a dead body and can also live on air and water alone for some days without any food.

Kunjal Kriya: Drink a large quantity of water and shake the abdominal portions. Contract the stomach and vomit the water. This exercise goes with the name 'Kunjal Kriya'.

Benefits:
Those who can do Antar-Dhauti need not go in for any purgative or laxative. They will never suffer from indigestion or constipation.

Bahar Dhauti can be made in the following ways: "Danta Dhauti" (cleaning the teeth), "Jihva Dhauti" (cleaning the tongue), 'Karna Dhauti" (cleaning the ears), "Mula Shodhana Dhauti" (cleaning the anus), face massage and face yoga, abhignya or self-massage.

3. NAULI

Nauli Kriya is intended for regenerating, invigorating, and stimulating the abdominal viscera and the gastrointestinal or alimentary system. For the practice of Nauli you should know the Uddiyana Bandha. Uddiyana can be done even in a sitting posture; but Nauli is generally done while standing.

Stage I: Do a strong and forcible expiration through the mouth and
keep the lungs completely empty. Contract and forcibly draw the abdominal
muscles towards the back. This is Uddiyana Bandha. This is the first stage
of Nauli. Uddiyana Bandha terminates in Nauli.
For practicing Nauli, stand up. Keep the right foot apart from the left. If you keep the feet close together, at times you may lose the balance and stumble down. Rest your hands on the thighs, thus making a slight curve of the back. Then do Uddiyana Bandha. Do this for one week before proceeding to the next stage.

Stage II: Now allow the center of the abdomen free by contracting the left and right side of the abdomen. You will have all the muscles in the center in a vertical line. This is called Madhyama Nauli. Keep it as long as you can with comfort. Do only this much for a few days.

Stage III: Here you should contract the right side of the abdomen and allow the left side free. This is called Vama Nauli. Again contract the left side muscles and allow the right side free. This is Dakshina Nauli. By having such gradual practices, you will understand how to contract the muscles of the central, left and right sides of the abdomen. You will also notice how they move from side to side. In this stage you will see the abdominal muscles only in the central, right, or the left side. Practice this stage for a week.

Stage IV: Keep the muscles in the center. Slowly bring to the right side and then to the left side in a circular way. Do this several times from the right to the left side and then do it in a reverse way from the left to the right side. You should always turn the muscles with a circular motion slowly. When you advance in the practice you can do it quickly; but you can derive full benefits of this Kriya when you do it very slowly and gradually. This last stage of Nauli will appear like 'churning' when the abdominal muscles are isolated and rotated from side to side. Beginners will feel slight pain in their abdomen in the first two or three attempts. They need not fear and stop the practice. The pain will vanish away in 2 or 3 days. When Nauli is demonstrated by the advanced Yogic student, the onlookers will be extremely surprised to look at the movements of the abdominal muscles. They will feel as if an engine is working in the abdominal factory.

When beginners want to do Dakshina Nauli, they should slightly bend towards the left side and contract the left muscles. When they want to do Vama Nauli, let them bend a little to the right side. In Madhyama Nauli,

push the entire muscles forward by contracting the two sides. This exercise is not at all possible for those who have a pot belly. They can also try by gradual slow practice. To be successful, they must exert hard and have rigorous practice for a long time. Those who have a tender body can very easily learn and perform this Kriya in a beautiful and efficient manner.

If the Yogic exercises are done in the right way with the right mental attitude, it will surely lead you to spiritual growth.

Benefits

Nauli Kriya eradicates chronic constipation, dyspepsia, and all other diseases of the gastrointestinal system. Nauli helps Basti Kriya also. The liver and pancreas are toned. The kidneys and other organs of the abdomen function properly. Nauli is a blessing to humanity. It is a sovereign specific 'uni-all' or an ideal 'pick- me-up.'

Contraindications: This kriya is not suitable for people with abdominal injuries, pregnant women, IBS patients, or during fever.

4. BASTI

'Basti' exercise is intended to serve the purpose of 'enema' to pass out the accumulation of feces from the intestinal canal.

There are two methods of basti:

1. Sthala Basti
2. Jala Basti

Sthala Basti

Sit on the ground and catch hold of your toes with the fingers. Do not bend the knees. This is exactly like the Paschimottanasana, but here you need not bring your head to the knees. Assuming this posture, churn the abdominal muscles, get the water in and then again churn the abdominal muscles and expel the water. It strengthens the ureter muscles.

Jala Basti

This is more effective than Sthala Basti. Take a small bamboo tube, five inches long. Lubricate one end of it with vaseline, oil, or soap. Sit in a tub of water or in a tank at knee- level of water in Utkatasana. Insert the bamboo tube about 2 or 3 inches into the anus. Contract the anus. Draw the water into the intestines slowly. Shake the abdominal muscles and expel the water.

Benefits:

It cures urinary troubles, dropsy, constipation, etc.

Contraindications: You should not do this every day and make it a habit. This is only for occasional use. Do this in the morning hours before taking meals. If you do not know how to draw in the water through the tube, then you can use the ordinary syringe that is available in the market. By the use of the bamboo, you will know the method of drawing water through the anus. But in the enema syringe, water is being pushed in by the help of air. That is only the difference but the result is the same in both the cases. By using the bamboo tube you can have mastery over the intestinal muscles by drawing in and pushing out the water at your command.

5. KAPALBHATI

Kapalabhatti is one of the most important Shatkarma practices for the purification of the skull and lungs. Though this is one of the Shat-Karmas (six purification processes), yet it is also a kind of pranayama too.

Method:

1. Sit in Padmasana or Siddhasana
2. Keep your hands on the knees
3. Perform Puraka (inhalation) that is very long and mild, and Rechaka (exhalation) that is too quick and forcible
4. In Kapalabhati, there is no Kumbhaka
5. Rechaka should be done forcibly and quickly by contracting the abdominal muscles with a backward push.
6. To start with, have only one expulsion per second.
7. In the beginning do 10 expulsions per round. Gradually increase 10 expulsions to each round until you get 120 expulsions for each round.

Benefits: It cleanses the respiratory system and nasal passages. It removes spasm in the bronchial tubes. Consequently asthma is relieved and cured also in course of time. Excess of kapha is cured by this practice. Impurities of the blood are thrown out. The circulatory and respiratory systems are toned to a considerable degree.

Benefits:

Shat-Karmas are intended for the purification of the body. When Nadis are impure, Kundalini cannot pass from the
Muladhara to the Sahasrara Chakra. Purification of Nadis is effected through pranayama. For details about Pranayama, please read the Pranayama section.

6. TRATAKA

'Trataka' is steady gazing at a particular point or object without winking. This is one of the six purification exercises and is mainly intended for developing concentration and mental focusing. It is very useful for the students of Hatha Yoga, Gyan Yoga, Bhakti Yoga, and Raja Yoga. There is no other effective method for the control of the mind.
Duration about 30 min.
I. Starting prayer (OM Sahana Vavatu.....)

II. Eye exercises

a) Up and down or vertical movements of the eyeballs
• Number of rounds: 10
• Palming: simple palming

b) Right and left or horizontal movement of the eyeballs
• Number of rounds: 10
• Palming: simple palming

c) Diagonal movement of eyeballs
• Right up and left down
• Left up and right down

- 10 rounds of each is to be performed followed by press and release
palming

d) Rotational or circular movement of eyeballs
- Clockwise
- Anti-clockwise
- 10 rounds of each followed by palming with constant pressure palming

III. Candle flame gazing (3 stages)

a) Focusing (on the whole flame)
- Palming: press and release palming

b) Intensive focusing (on the tip of the wick)
- Palming: palming with constant pressure

Indications for candle flame gazing steps a and b
- *Continuously gazing at the flame*
- *No blinking or winking*
- *Smooth and effortless gazing*
- *Use your will power and ignore watering or irritation in the eyes*
- *Gazing for 30 – 60 sec*

c) De-focusing
Indications for candle flame gazing step c
- *Focus on the whole flame for a few seconds*
- *Slowly defocus your attention by expanding your vision, i.e. de-focused look at the flame*
- *See the aura around the flame, gradually becoming bigger and bigger*
- *Also see the small-small light particles around the flame*

- *Enjoy this expansive state for about a minute*
- *Again focus on the whole flame for a few seconds*
- *Close your eyes and visualize the "after-image" of the flame between*
- *eyebrows*
- *As the image disappears, go for palming with Bhramari (5 rounds)*

VII. Silence: At the end, sit quietly for some time.

VIII. Closing prayer (Asato ma sadgamaya....)

Tips for the practitioners:

1. Remove glasses, wrist watches, belts and be comfortable in the
posture
2. Sit with your head, neck, and spine upright
3. Always open the eyes with a few blinks
4. During Jyoti (light) trataka when you open the eyes, don't look at
the flame right away; start looking at the floor and then slowly bring your gaze upon the flame
6. During eye exercise, you must not move your head. Only eyeballs
move
7. During Trataka practices, try not to blink or move the eyeballs in
any direction
8. During palming, don't let the fingers touch or press the eyeballs. The palms, not the fingers, cover the eyes
9. Do palming very slowly and with deep breathing and awareness

10. Palms are placed in such a way that there is complete darkness to the eyes

11. The facial muscles, eyebrows, and eyelids should remain totally relaxed – a beautiful smile in the face.

12. Trataka should be performed after asanas and pranayamas.

13. Trataka must be practiced on a steady flame.

14. The practitioner should always avoid strain to the eyes.

Benefits of Trataka:

- Physical

1. Helps with reducing and removing eye strain by improving the stamina of muscles and deep relaxation to them

2. It makes eyes clear, bright, and radiant

3.

It cleanses the tear glands and purifies the optical system

- Therapeutic

1. Observatory refraction errors get corrected as the external eye muscles improve

2. Strengthens the ciliary muscles (short and long sightedness are reduced)

3. Balances the nervous system, relieving nervous tension, anxiety, depression, and insomnia.

4. Those who suffer from insomnia and mental tension should perform this practice of gazing continuously or 10-15 minutes before going to sleep at night

- Spiritual

1. Helps to develop concentration and improves memory
2. Helps to develop a strong willpower.
3. It is an excellent preparation for meditation.

Limitations and contraindications:
1. Glaucoma patients should avoid or do under proper guidance.
2. Epileptics should avoid candle flame gazing. They can, however, choose a totally steady object to gaze on.
3. People with eye infection should avoid it
4. In case of burning sensation in the eyes or headache, one should avoid this practice.

Similar Practices:
1. Keep the picture of Lord Krishna, Rama, Narayana, or Devi in front of you. Look at it steadily without winking. Gaze at the head; then at the body; then at the legs. Repeat the same process again and again. When your mind calms down, look at a particular place only. Be steady till tears begin to flow. Then close the eyes and mentally visualize the picture.
2. Gaze on a black dot on a white wall or draw a black mark on a piece of white paper and hang it on the wall in front of you.
3. Draw the picture OM on a piece of paper and have it before your seat. Do trataka on it.
4. Lie down on an open terrace and gaze at a particular bright star or on the full moon. After some time, you will see different colors of lights. Again some time later, you will see only a particular star throughout, and all other

surrounding stars will disappear. When you gaze at the moon, you will see only a bright moon on a black background. At times you will see a huge mass of light all around you. When gazing becomes more intense, you can also see two or three moons of the same size and at times you cannot see any moon at all even though your eyes may be wide open.

5. Select at random any place in the open sky in the morning or evening hours and gaze at the sky steadily. You will get new inspirations.

6. Look at a mirror and gaze at the pupil of your eye.

7. Some people do trataka at the space between the two eyebrows or at the tip of the nose. Even while walking, one can do trataka at the tip of the nose.

8. Advanced students can do trataka at the inner Chakras (Padmas). Muladhara, Anahata, Ajna and Sahasrara are the important centers for trataka.

9. Keep a ghee-lamp before you and gaze at the flames. Some astral entities give Darshan through the flames.

10. Very few Yogis do trataka of the sun. It requires the help of an experienced person by their side. They begin to gaze on the rising sun and after gradual practice they do trataka on the sun even in the midday. They get some special Siddhis (psychic powers) by this practice. All are not fit for this Sadhana. All the first 9 exercises will suit everyone and they are harmless. The last one, sun-gazing should not be attempted until you get the help of an experienced person / teacher.

More instructions:

When you do the Trataka in your meditation room, sit in your favorite asana (posture), Siddhasana or Padmasana. At other times you can do it in a standing or sitting posture. Trataka can be profitably done even when you walk. As you walk along the streets, do not look hither and thither. Gaze at the tip of the nose or toes. No particular asana is required for this Sadhana.

When you gaze at a picture, it is trataka. When you close your eyes and mentally visualize the picture, it is Saguna Dhyana (meditation with form). When you associate the attributes of God such as omnipresence, omnipotence, omniscience, purity, perfection, etc., the name and the form of the object of trataka will automatically disappear and you will enter into Nirguna Dhyana (abstract meditation).

Do trataka for two minutes to start with. Then cautiously increase the period. Do not be impatient. Gradual steady practice is required. Gazing at a spot even for three full hours continuously counts for nothing, if the mind is wandering. The mind also must be on the spot. Then only you will advance in this practice and attain many psychic powers.

Those who cannot gaze steadily for a second in spite of several attempts need not worry much. They can close their eyes and gaze at an imaginary spot in the space between the two eyebrows.

Those who have very weak eye capillaries should do trataka after closing their eyes on any imaginary spot within or without. Do not tax your eyes by over-practicing. When you feel tired, close your eyes and keep your mind on the object of trataka. When you sit and do trataka, do not shake the body.

Trataka improves eyesight. Many who have had some eye troubles have realized immense benefits from trataka.

Going beyond one's own power and gazing at the sun without any help may produce serious troubles. For gazing at the sun you must have your guide by your side. The Guru will prescribe some oil to rub on your head to avoid such serious troubles and to cool the system. You should apply honey to your eyes at night when you practice sun gazing.

The same object of gazing will appear as something else during the practice. You will have many other visions. Different people have different experiences. You will not even believe certain things when others tell you of their experiences. Trataka alone cannot give you all Siddhis. After the control of the mind, when it becomes steady, you will have to manipulate the mind by prescribed methods for the attainment of powers. Therefore the powers that are obtained by this practice may vary in different persons. It depends upon the further training of the mind in a particular way.

Through the practice of trataka:

1. Diseases of the eyes are removed.
2. Eyesight improves.
3. Many have thrown away their spectacles after taking this practice.
4. Willpower is developed.
5. Vikshepa (sorrow) is destroyed.
6. Steadies' the mind.
7. Clairvoyance, thought reading, psychic cure and other Siddhis are
obtained very easily.

Even though you may claim to be a student of Gyan Yoga or Bhakti Yoga, you can take this practice. It is a very effective and powerful remedy for a wandering mind. It undoubtedly prepares the mind for perfect Dhyana and Samadhi. This is assuredly a means for the end. You must ascend the yogic ladder or staircase step by step. Several people have been benefited by this useful exercise. Select any one of the methods that suits you best and realize the spiritual benefits. Do this for one month regularly to experience the full benefits.

Shankhaprakshalana

As per Yoga and Ayurveda, if your intestine is upset, your life will be upset because one of the secrets of physical health resides in the large intestine. One of the main causes of various diseases and senility is the accumulation of toxins in the organism by autointoxication. The intoxication is extremely dangerous, the poisons infiltrate through the walls of the large intestine (colon and rectum) spreading through the entire organism. Constipation or irregular bowel movements become common problems. The evacuation, even on a daily basis, does not mean that your intestine is totally clean. Intestines form putrid fermentations, whose toxins spread in the entire organism. Only in the United States, every 9 minutes a person dies because of colorectal cancers (colon and rectum forming the large intestine).

The diseases deriving directly from auto-intoxication are: Constipation, anemia, cirrhosis, rheumatism, dysentery, heart problems, skin diseases, bad mouth smell, kidney stones, insomnia, and sciatica.

Results of irregular bowel movements

- Ulcers
- Cancer
- Bad breath
- Kidney stones
- Insomnia
- Depression
- Irritability
- Hysteria
- Sciatica
- Varicose
- Liver intoxications
- Chronic or acute appendicitis

- Anemia
- Skin eruptions of different natures
- Painful periods

Our Yogis of ancient times gifted us a great and ideal method of cleansing toxins, called as Shank Prakshalana (or Varisara Dhauti). Shankh in Sanskrit means conch. Conch has the similarity of the sinuous digestive system with the corridors of the shell; therefore in English it means "Conch Shell Cleansing". To a great surprise, this technique is not found in the majority of yoga scriptures in detail as it was kept as a secret for a very long time.

Technique

For this cleansing, warm water added with salt is used. Water reaches the stomach, where, by simple movements, washes the entire surface of the large intestine on its way out. The yogic exercise stops when the water comes out as clean as it enters. This process doesn't involve any major difficulties or efforts. It is recommended to anyone, on the condition that the technique is correctly done.

How is it done?

1. Heat drinking water until lukewarm.

2. Add a dosage of 15-16 grams of salt per liter of water, which is

equivalent to a spoonful of salt for every liter.

3. The water is to be salty; otherwise, it will not reach the colon. It will

be absorbed passing the mucous membrane and will be evacuated

as urine.

4. Capacity of the water cup can be 250 ml.

5. While performing these steps, the toilet should be available nearby.

Preferred Timing

The best moment for Shankh Prakshalana is early in the morning, on an empty stomach. These techniques may last for more than an hour or 90 minutes. After this process, on that day one should not perform asanas, exercise, or work hard physically.

The Procedure

Follow step by step to get better results:

- Drink a cup of warm salty water (temperature like a warm soup).
- Immediately afterwards, perform a set of yogic movements.
- Drink another cup of water.
- Follow another set of similar movements.
- Continue this procedure and exercise until 6 cups of drinking water.
- After the 6th cup, you should go to the toilet.
- Normally, the first evacuation appears quickly. Even if it gets delayed, wait till it happens.
- Once the first evacuation happens, the rest will follow automatically.
- After the use of the toilet, the anus is washed with warm water. It should be dried and anointed with either oil or ointment. This will avoid rashes caused by the salt.
- After going to the toilet the first time, you must drink again a cup of lukewarm salty water.
- Perform the exercises and go back to the toilet, each time, a new evacuation will take place.
- The procedure of drinking salty water and then performing a set of exercises and going

to the toilet will continue until the water comes out as clear as when it enters the stomach.

- This may continue until 10 to 14 glasses of salty water, more than that being seldom required.
- Drink 3 more cups of plain warm water
- Perform Vamana dhauti. This will close the siphon. Completely empty the stomach.

For patients with severe constipation or over anxiety, if the evacuation does not happen, follow the following:

- After drinking 6 glasses, if you feel that the contents of the stomach are not passing to the intestine and causing a sensation of overloading and nausea, then still continue to ease the process.
- Press firmly on the abdomen with the hands doing the abdominal massage (Sahaj Agnisara Dhauti) or perform Pawanmuktasana, apart from the indicated exercises.
- In worst cases, if water does not leave at all, perform any of the following solutions:
- One should trigger the evacuation eventually by an enema with 1⁄2 liter of water
- Make Vamana dhauti or Kunjal Kriya (empty stomach by tickling the base of the tongue with three fingers of the right hand to start the vomit reflex).
- Do nothing; let the water be evacuated normally, progressively, as urine.
- After doing the exercise, it is absolutely necessary to rest to avoid the cold.

After Shank Prakshalana, it is necessary to follow the following steps respecting oneself:

- Eat Khichdi within 1 hour. Do not let the digestive tube empty for more than an hour.
- The first meal will be Khichdi (white rice) boiled in water. It should be well boiled so as it melts in the mouth. First Khichdi should be made with good butter.
- Do not boil Khichdi with milk.
- For the next 24 hours, do not drink milk or eat yogurt and other dairy products and avoid acid foods, drinks, raw fruits, and vegetables.
- Bread and other soft vegetarian meals are allowed after 3 days.
- No yoga asana or exercises for the next 24 hrs and only mild activities, can re-start activities after 24 hrs.
- The ejection may be after 24 or 36 hours. This may be yellow- golden, just as that of a little baby.
- Resist thirst at least until after the first meal, otherwise, you will continue to go to the toilet nonstop.
- This technique can be done at least twice a year during the change of seasons.

Benefits

- Total evacuation of the encrusted sediments in the mucous membrane of the large intestine including parasites.
- The illusion that one is not constipated, can be seen in their excrement peels of fruit, seeds, hair, etc., all of these being encrusted in the colon or rectum for months or even years.

- These filths are eliminated, the danger of intoxication due to their presence as permanently distilled toxins are being suspended.
- The benefits will not appear immediately, but after 2-3 days, by the freshness of breath, better sleep, disappearance of rashes and pimples on the face or the body.
- Disappearance of bodily bad odors.
- Skin may become lighter, shinier, and magnetic.
- It strengthens the immune system.
- Helps to relieve arthritis and purifies the blood.
- Liver is deeply stimulated.
- The pancreas secretes more insulin.
- Balance the body weight.
- Good for allergies, fatigue, acidity, and gas.
- Recharges the whole body, removes blockages from the nadis and purifies the chakras.

Contraindications: These contraindications are not absolute. In India, there are cases of dysentery and many diseases are healed by Shank Prakshalana in Yogi's hospital.

- If severe stomach ulcer or acute illness or fever, one must refrain and wait to heal before practicing.
- If the digestive imbalances like dysentery, diarrhea, acute colitis, acute appendicitis or serious illnesses such as intestinal tuberculosis or cancer, one must consult a teacher before doing so.

- It should not be practiced during pregnancy or menstruation, big kidney or gallbladder stone, weak kidneys, chronic diabetes, or hernia.

Yogic Kriya/Yogic Movements for Shankh Prakshalana:

Introduction
1. Water passes through the digestive tube to exit with the help of these yogic movements.
2. Repeat each movement 5 times in each direction in a rapid rhythm.
3. On an average, each session should be about 3 minutes maximum.

▶ First Kriya: Tritanka Tadasana
1. Stand on your feet 30-cm apart.
2. Lift up your arms and straighten them.
3. The fingers interlocked and the palms facing up.
4. Straighten the back.
5. Stretch your body upwards.
6. Breathe normally.
7. Without twisting, first bend towards left, then without stopping bend towards the right.
8. Repeat 5 times in each direction.
9. This movement can open the stomach towards the duodenum and small
Intestine.

▶ Second Kriya: Twisting
This movement will help in the movement of water towards the small
intestine.
1. Stand with your feet 30 cm apart.

2. The right arm is stretched horizontally and the left arm is bent until
the forefinger and the thumb touch the right clavicle.
3. A rotation of the body is performed pulling the straightened right
arm towards the back as far as possible.
4. Gaze at the tip of the fingers.
5. Change the direction and perform the movement on the other side.
6. This double movement rotation will be repeated 5 times.

▶ Third Kriya: Bhujangasana Twisting
Water will continue to advance further in the small intestine and will
enter the large intestine with the help of the following movements:
1. Lay down on your belly in Bhujangasana (Cobra pose)
2. Spread your legs apart about 2 inches.
3. Only the palms and the toes will be touching the floor.
4. When your head is up, then twist the head, the shoulders, and the trunk until you can see the opposite heel.
5. If you start the turn towards the right, then look at the left heel.
6. Return to the initial position and start again on the other side.
7. Breathe normally.
8. This double movement is to be repeated 5 times, making a total of 10 rotations

▶ Fourth Kriya: Hunkers Twisting

Due to this kriya, water will reach the extremity of the small intestine and must be evacuated through the colon. It is comfortable to anyone except for people who suffer with knee problems.

1. Sit on your feet in Hunkers' position.
2. With the feet spread apart 2 inches and head facing the exterior of the calf, the arms are placed on the knees
3. The left knee is placed on the floor in front of the opposite leg. The palms push the right calf towards the left side and the left calf towards the right. This will compress half of the abdomen and press on the colon.
4. Look back as much as possible, turning the head to accentuate the torsion of the trunk and to increase the pressure over the abdomen.
5. It is necessary to first start by placing the left knee on the floor to compress the right side of the abdomen
6. To be executed 5 times (8 torsions)

In case the fourth movement cannot be executed, the replacing variant will be done.
Persons with problems in performing the fourth kirya can perform an alternate method.

1. Sit on the floor with one leg straight and another bending from the knee in Vakrasana.
2. The right leg is bent and placed over the left one.
3. Place the right palm on the sole of the right feet and stretch the left
arm behind the back for support.
4. Turn the trunk as much as possible towards the left, looking back.
5. Perform the same procedure from the other side.
6. Breathing is normal.

7. There will be 5 rounds on each side, a total of 10 on both sides

Chakra Yoga and Kundalini Awakening

Chakras

Chakra is a Sanskrit name. It means wheel. It refers to energy points in our body
Chakras are thought to be spinning disks of energy that should stay open and aligned. Chakras correspond to a bundle of nerves organs and areas of our energetic body that affect our emotional and physical well-being
Some say we have 140 different chakras, but there are seven main chakras that run along our spine. These are the chakras that most of us talk about. So each of these chakras have a corresponding number, color and specific area from the sacrum to the crown of the head.

THE ROOT CHAKRA - 7th chakra

The location of the root chakra is the base of the spine. Moola bandha. The Moola bandha conserves and energizes the root chakra. The color of this chakra is red. The physical identity of this chakra is stability and grounding.
A block to root chakra can manifest as physical issues like arthritis, constipation and bladder problems, a block in this chakra can also result in emotionally feeling insecure about finance or our basic needs. When it's in alignment and open we

will feel grounded and secure both physically and emotionally.

THE SACRAL CHAKRA - 6th chakra

The location of the sacral chakra is just below the belly button and above the public bone. The color is orange. It is also called swadisthan chakra. This chakra is about sexuality, pleasure and creativity. Some issues with this chakra can be seen as problems associated with organs like urinary tract infections, lower back pain and impotence. Emotionally this chakra is connected to our feelings of self - worth and even more specially our self - worth around pleasure, security and creativity.

THE MANIPURA CHAKRA - 5th chakra

The Solar plexus chakra, the location of the manipura chakra, is at the upper abdomen in the stomach area. The color of this chakra is yellow. This chakra is about self - esteem and confidence. Sometimes. If we have blockage in this 3rd chakra, it's often experienced through digestive issues like ulcers, heartburn, eating disorders and indigestion. This is the chakra for our personal power because it's related to our self – esteem and self confidence

THE HEART CHAKRA - ANAHATA CHAKRA - .4th chakra

The location of this chakra is in the center of the chest just above the heart. Sometimes in our class we also call it the heart center. The color of this chakra is green. This chakra is about love and compassion. A block in the heart chakra can manifest in our physical health as heart problems, asthma and weight issues. Blocks are often seen more clearly with the people's action. The people with heart chakra blocks often put themselves first to others detriment.

The heart chakra is in the middle of the seven chakras. So it bridges the gap between our upper and lower chakras. It also represents our ability to love and connect to others. When this chakra is out of alignment, it can make us feel lonely, sad, insecure and isolated

THE THROAT CHAKRA - Vishuddhi Chakra - 3rd chakra

The location of the throat chakra is in the throat. The color of this chakra is blue. This chakra is more about communication. This chakra is connected to our ability to communicate verbally. Voice and throat problems as well as any problems surrounding that area such as the teeth, gums and mouth can indicate a blockage. Blocks in the alignment of this chakra can be seen by dominating conversation and speaking without thinking and having trouble speaking your mind. When this chakra is in alignment you will speak and listen with compassion and feel confident when you speak because you know that you are being true to yourself with your words

THE THIRD EYE CHAKRA - AJNA CHAKRA 2nd chakra

The location of the Ajna chakra is between the eyes of the forehead. The color of this chakra is indigo. It's about imagination and intuition. This chakra is basically located on the head. The blockages can be manifested as headache issues with sight or concentration and hearing problems. The person who has trouble listening to reality or who is not in touch with their intuition. When this chakra is open and aligned people will follow their intuition and be able to see the big picture.

THE CROWN CHAKRA - SAHASRARA - 1st chakra

The location of this chakra is on the top of the head. The color of this chakra is violet or white. This chakra is about awareness and intelligence. The crown chakra is linked to every other chakra, so it affects not just all the organs but also our brain and nervous systems. It is considered the chakra of enlightenment and represents our connection to our life's purpose and spirituality. Those who have blockage of the crown chakra may seem narrow-minded and stubborn. When this chakra is open, it is thought to help keep all the other chakras open and to bring the person bliss and enlightenment. These are all energetic centers of the body that correspond to feelings. When you often deal with blockages, other blockages may pop up. In the chakra system these patterns have specific terms and there are recommended treatments.
Chakra balancing and realignment: This can be many things including
  - Yoga
  - Meditation

- Chakra cleansing through pranayama
- Certain types of body works
- Music

NADIS

We have the ida (moon channel) and pingala nadi (sun channel). All the chakras are with the sushumna nadi; the middle path. The sushumna nadi is located at the center of the spinal cord. Though physically we cannot see it, it starts from the base of the spine at the muladhara chakra. From the muladhara chakra, it passes through the spine and completes its journey in the crown sahasrara chakra at the crown of the head

- Nadis are like invisible flow of energy
- We have 72000 nadis. The yogis and Ayurveda scriptures say there are 72000 nadis present in the body
- Once a yogi attains success with regulation of the nadis, he gets access to his own body
- Through the subtle body, one can also see these nadis through their inner vision
- In our body we have two opposite energies like positive and negative. These are represented by ida nadi and pingala nadi
- The sushumna nadi which flows through the center is the most important

Ida Nadi

- The ida nadi starts from the muladhara chakra. This nadi is from the left side of the body and also the left side from the sushumna nadi crossing each chakra. This nadi completes its journey into the ajna third eye chakra from the left side. Even though it is invisible yet it is very powerful

- Ida nadi represented and processes passive introvert and feminine characteristics which is also known as chandra nadi; moon channel

Pingala Nadi

- Originates from the right side of muladhara chakra. This nadi travels through the right hand side of the body and crosses each chakra in a serpentine manner. This nadi terminates at the ajna chakra and terminates at the right side
- Pingala nadi represents and processes active extrovert and masculine characteristics. It is also known as surya nadi; sun channel

We perform many activities every day. These activities are affected by the change in the flow within the nadis. These flows change from one nadi to another in about every 60 - 90 minutes. But with some yogic practices and techniques the yogi can alter this flow as per their wish. For example, your pingala nadi is more active, but at that time you need to perform mental work. You can change the flow to ida nadi through yogic practices like chandrabedhana pranayama so that you have more energy available for mental works

KUNDALINI YOGA

Yoga that involves chanting singing movements
This is a spiritual energy that's located at the base of your spine
As kundalini yoga awakens this energy, it is supposed to enhance your awareness and help you to move past your ego

Characteristics of kundalini yoga
- Also called yoga if awareness
- Kundalini yoga is associated with yogi bhajans
- The term kundalini comes from Sanskrit
- It comes from the name kundal which means circular
- It also refers to a curled snake
- Kundalini energy sits at the base of your spine. Kundalini yoga is practiced to activate this energy which allows it to move up and through the chakras along your spine
- Kundalini yoga defines yoga chakras which are the 7 energy centers in your body. The chakras are:
  Root
  Sacral
  Naval or solar
  Heart
  Throat
  Third eye
  Crown
- As Kundalini energy arises its believed to balance these chakras and continue to your spiritual wellness

- The regular practice of Kundalini yoga leads to spiritual Alignment - Kundalini awakening

How is it different?

If we compare with other forms of yoga, Kundalini yoga is a more spiritual practice and it still involves physical movement but they are not the primary focus
- This is different from hatha and vinyasa yoga
- Kundalini yoga is more precise and repetitive
- But other types of yoga flow is with your breath
- Kundalini yoga combines chanting singing movements and breathing

Kundalini Yoga consists of 6 main components

1) Opening chant
Every class begins with opening chant

2) Pranayama or warm ups ' breathing and sometimes movements to stretch your spine

3) Kriya
Kriya is sequence of postures Pranayama mudra sounds and meditation

4) Relaxation
This allows your body and mind to observe the effect of kriya

5) Meditation
It's for more awareness

6) Closing chant
The class will close with closing chant

The benefits
1. Stress and anxiety relief
2. Spiritual enlightenment

With the help of kundalini yoga you become more spiritually connected with yourself and with others
It increases creativity energy and internal peace

Kundalini yoga safe
Kundalini Yoga is like all yoga should be practiced with safety in mind
If someone has breathing issues joint pain or injury or balance problems and for the pregnant
- Here Kundalini Yoga is more Spiritual than other types of yoga
- Other types of yoga flow with the breath
- The purpose is to promote spiritual enlightenment

Basic Kundalini yoga pose for beginners

- Lotus pose
- Cobra pose

Some Signs of rising Kundalini Shakti

- Jumping
- Trembling
- Drowsiness
- Ecstatic feeling- Ananda
- Shaking of the body
- Laughing

- Crying
- Sounds
- Fear
- Breath becomes extremely slow
- Inner flow of feeling rising currents of prana
- Divine sounds om starts automatically
- Powerful vibrations movements
- Extreme lightness emptiness of body
- Contraction
- Body rotations twisting
- Faster or Extreme slow walk
- Disturbed meditative movement
- Louder sound
- Uncontrollable movements of limbs
- Automatically third eye activates
- Sambhavi mudra becomes easier
- Divine vision
- Divine taste
- Divine sounds can be experienced
- Musical sound with the unknown language and also maybe poetry may start
- Feel like drunk of divinity and no attachment to the world

Removing Knots (granthis) during the process. That is very important for attaining the goal

We have three knots or granthis
1. Brahma granthi at the base of the spine which represents Brahma
2. Vishnu granthi at the throat which represents Vishnu
3. Rudra granthi at the third eye between both the eyebrows which represents Shiva

Awakening of Kundalini Shakti is
  - Freedom
  - Purity
  - Bliss
  - During Kundalini, awakening or initiation can happen which is sometimes beyond common understanding. This happening is not controlled nor with effort or choice
  - It's called Leela or divine play or leela

Try to do more meditation relaxation chanting Mantras
You need to give more time for kundalini practice.

MEDITATION, YOGA NIDRA AND SAMADHI

Meditation

Meditation refers to a technique of focusing the mind inwards and becoming aware of the present moment. It is also called mindfulness meditation. Meditation can also be done by focusing on a particular object, thought or activity. In Ashtanga yoga, meditation falls within 'Pratyahara', 'Dharana', 'Dhyana' and also 'Samadhi'. Meditation helps in achieving a mentally and emotionally calm and stable state of mind. Meditation helps to get rid of fear and anxiety and enables a better state of health and wellbeing.

Meditation is practiced easily and effortlessly and can be done for 10 to 15 minutes two times in a day. Clearing of the mind is not the objective of meditation and the mind should be free to wander without inhibitions during meditation. As the practitioner does meditation regularly and with normal intentions; an inner peace, emotional balance and a spiritual connection is found.

Technique:
Take this moment to find a comfortable place, seated; grounded. Let us take this opportunity to find a peaceful presence from within. Driving our awareness inwards as we close our eyes, simply focus on the inhales and the exhales. Breathe in and breathe out
Setting an intention to breathe in life force energy, breathe in and feel the energy within our heart. Know that you are worthy to receive your heart's

desires and live a beautiful life guided through love, peace and gratitude

Breathe in and let go

Allow yourself to settle in within yourself deeper and deeper

Feel the sensations and the movement of your breath and you inhale and exhale

Feel the cool air moving in as you breathe in and the warm air moving out as you breathe out.

Allow the breath to ground you and guide you to a closer connection to your vast an infinite potential

Look within yourself, feel the movement of your breath and notice the happenings, desires and feelings within you

Inhale and exhale as you sink deeper into stillness

Let go and surrender to stillness

Keep your present awareness on your breath and set an intention ' I am fulfilled, happy, peaceful and smiling'

Repeat this intention at your own pace silently in your mind (5 minutes)

As you start releasing your intentions, bring your focus back to your breath. Inhale and exhale

Feel the sensations and energy within you. Gently and slowly open your eyes

The Nadis, Pranayama and Meditation

Nadis are invisible energy channels in the subtle body and are said to enable the flow of prana or life force energy which is required for all living things. The nadis are said to go through the spinal cord and the chakras, Asanas, pranayama and chanting allow the energy to travel through the body through the nadis. Our body consists of 7200 nadis that spring from 3 basic nadis: the ida, the pingala and the sushumna nadi.

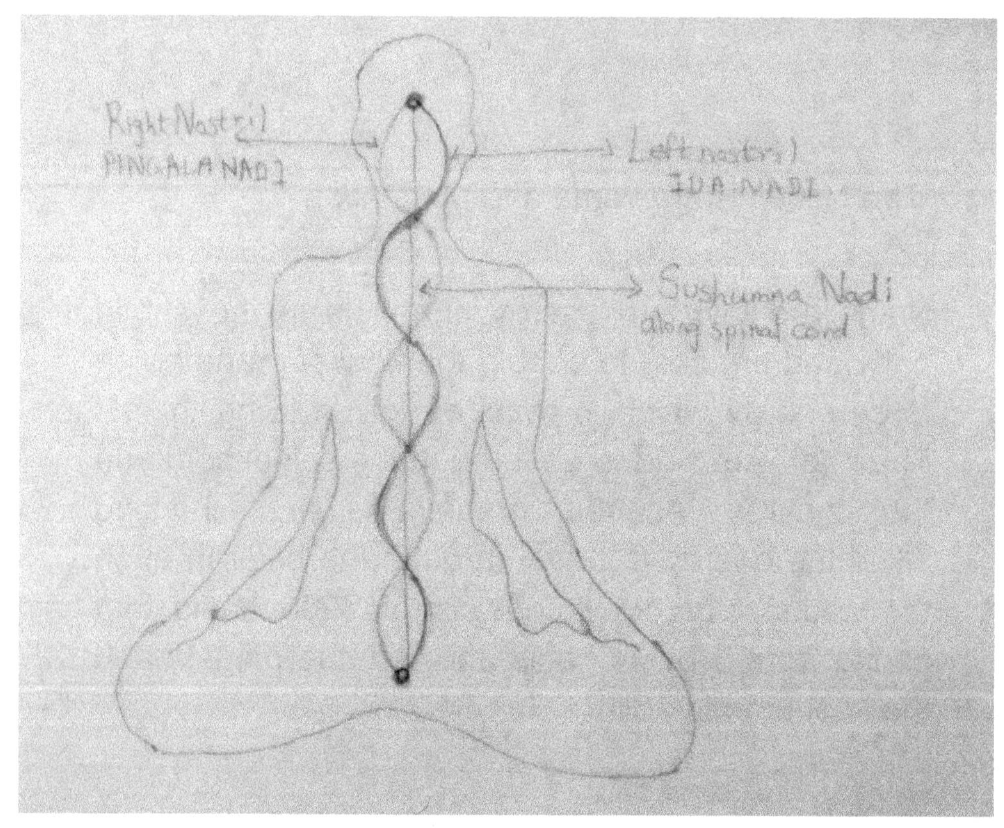

Nadis, Suryabedhan, Chandrabedhan

1. **Ida Nadi** - moon - cool- left

The left nostril belongs to the moon. Its name is ida nadi'. The Ida nadi gives you more coolness and makes your body calmer. The Ida nadi also refers to 'Chandrabedhi'.

Chandrabedhan

In Sanskrit Chandra means moon and bedhan means revealing the secret of moon. The complementary practice is Suryabedhan which refers to the sun. Concentration of the breath into the left nostril, Ida nadi is the channel which is responsible for more calm and receptive energy. It can also be performed by closing the right nostril and inhaling and exhaling from the left side.

Benefits: Chandrabedhan pranayama can be used to relax our body and mind and it also provides relief from anxiety, insomnia and for cooling the body and relax and peace of mind

Therapeutic benefits:
It helps alleviate migraine, allergies and skin problems

Technique: Sit in any comfortable pose back straight, relax the whole body, mind keep eyes closed.
- Inhale and exhale from the left nostril
- Inhale from left nostril and exhale from right nostril

2. **Pingala nadi**- sun - hot - right

Right nostril belongs to the sun. Its name is pingala nadi. When you inhale from the right nostril it gives you warmth. It gives you more hotness inside your body

Suryabhedana - inhale from the right after sitting comfortably relaxed

Technique:

1) Close your eyes relax the whole body and when the body is comfortable and still then relax, hold the breath for a few minutes until it becomes more slow and deep
2) After that close the left nostril with the ring finger and inhale slowly and deeply through the right nostril and at the end of inhalation, close both the nostrils
3) Retain the breath (you can with jalandhara bandha and mula bandha)
4) Exhale after releasing the bandhas (first release the mula bandha and then release the jalandhara bandha)
5) When the head is upright then exhale same side or the left side. Every inhalation should be from the right nostril
6) Duration: 10 rounds is sufficient. After that when the practice becomes more comfortable and easy, you can increase upto 10 - 15 minutes
7) Slowly increase the length of the retention
   - In the beginning ratio can be 1:1;1
   - Afterwards you can increase it to 1:2:2
   - Later you can increase it to 1:4: 2

Precautions

- Never practice Suryabedhan pranayama after food as it disturbs the natural forces of energy
- This is a very powerful pranayama. This pranayama may cause imbalance in the breathing cycle if you perform more than 30 minutes

Contra indications: Persons suffering from heart disease, hypertension, and high blood pressure should not perform Surya Bhedana pranayama

Benefits
- This practice creates heat in the body and it makes the mind more alert and this is an excellent pre meditation pranayama
- It is also useful in low blood pressure

3. **Sushumna nadi**: This is the central nadi that runs up the length of the spinal cord and through each of the chakras.it connects the base chakra to the crown chakra. 'Sushum' means; good' or 'virtuous' and 'mna' means 'to think' and this is where the kundalini awakening takes place. It connotes a 'joyful mind' or 'most gracious mind'.

4. **Anulom Vilom nadi shodhana-** Nadis are invisible energy channels or energy nerves in our body and shodan means purification. Nadi shodan means a pranayama which purifies our nadis. As per yogic science we have 72000 nadis in the human body, some we call as purush. The structure and operation of the human body is like a large city of 72000

streets which we need to keep clean. This can be done easier with the nadi shodan pranayama. Some yogis also call this pranayama as anulom vilom. Anulom means straight and vilom means reverse. In this technique the duration of inhalation and exhalation is controlled.

Technique: Sit in sukhasana or padmasana with your head, neck and spine in a straight line and keep the left hand in chi or gyan mudra on the left knee. Make nasika mudra with the right hand and close your eyes. Begin inhaling from the left nostril and retain the breath inside, then close the left nostril and open the right nostril. Slowly exhale from the right nostril and then inhale through the right nostril and retain and then exhale through the left nostril. The whole procedure we should do with awareness.

There are several ways to perform alternate nostril breathing. Each involves a unique rhythm of inhaling purak, internal retention 'antar kumbhaka' and exhaling hand retaining 'bhayaya kumbhaka'.

The purpose of the pranayama is to clean and purify the nadis

Ratio and timing: After a few days of practice, if there are no difficulties, you can increase the length of inhalation and exhalation by one count

    a. The maintenance of a strict ratio during inhalation, kumbhaka and exhalation is important. The ratio will change as the ability to hold the breath for longer periods of time. So after mastering the ratio of 1:1:1; increase the ratio to 1:1:2. For example inhale for a count of 5 then perform internal kumbhaka for a count of 5 and then exhale for a count of 10

b. After some weeks of practice when this ratio has been mastered, increase the ratio to 1:2:2.

After mastering the ratio of 1:2:2, increase the count by adding 1 unit to the inhalation, 2 units to the retention and 2 units to the exhalation

So here the count of 1 round is 6:12:12 or 7:14:14

Contraindications: Do not force the breath and holding breath to the best of your abilities for effective cleansing of nadis by nadi shodan

Benefits: Balances the nervous system and energetic channels and it brings balance to the mind. When the flow of prana is equal in both ida and pingala nadi, it can begin to enter sushumna nadi. Sushumna nadi is the central channel which allows kundalini energy to rise. All the chakras is on the sushumna

Yoga Nidra - Divine Sleep

Yoga Nidra is a deep and holistic relaxation technique in which muscular, emotional and mental tensions are eased and enables a natural positive mindset. Being scientifically based, yoga nidra is 'dynamic 'or 'psychic' sleep in which you learn to relax consciously. Yoga Nidra originated from the Tantras and has many benefits.

Benefits of Yoga Nidra

- Yoga Nidra gives a real positive direction to our life
- Eliminates the root cause of all negativities like stress related disorders and ailments like hypertension, depression, insomnia, asthma and digestive disorders which drain our life energy
- It trains the mind to delve into the subconscious and unconscious mind which are the most powerful forces in the human being and have immeasurable powers.
- It provides the key to access these powerful forces in the latent realms of the mind and to gain knowledge, cure diseases, increase creativity, and to realize one's true self

- A single hour of yoga nidra is as restful and refreshing as a four hours of conventional sleep.

Other benefits:

- The results are quicker and more reliable and permanent
- Improved quality of sleep
- Increased work efficiency
- Awakening of the psychic body and the astral plane
- Learning anything becomes very quick

Sankalpa

Sankalpa is a means in yoga nidra. It is a resolution, which you make for yourself during each practice. Anything in life can fail you but not your sankalpa. Therefore, sankalpa is a powerful way of reshaping your personality and giving a new direction in life along positive lines.

When the conscious mind-body is in deep relaxation, at that time, whatever sankalpa or- resolution you make, will get fulfilled.

The sankalpa is a short mental statement which is impressed on the subconscious mind when it is receptive and sensitive to autosuggestions during yoga nidra. Sankalpa is a determination to become something or to do something in your life. The sankalpa has to be made when you are not intellectually active, but when your mind is calm and quiet. Sankalpa is a seed which you create and then sow in the soil of your mind. When the mind is clear, the sankalpa grows well.

This deep and powerful seed will eventually manifest itself again and again at a conscious level and bring about the desired transformations in your personality and your life.

No personality is beyond reformation through yoga nidra. No fear or obsession is so deep rooted that it cannot be changed by the sankalpa made during yoga nidra.

However, the purpose of sankalpa is not to fulfill desires but to create strength in the structure of the mind. A sankalpa should only be made when one understands its real purpose and meaning.

Some examples of Sankalpa:
- I am energetic.
- I am the embodiment of inner peace.
- I receive and accept help when I need it.
- I am successful in all that I undertake.
- I am financially free.
- I am loving and loved

Y

o
g
a

N
i
d
r
a

S
c
r
i
p
t

Preparation: Get ready for Yoga Nidra, a complete physical, emotional and mental relaxation for you. Lie down on your mat in savasana with your head facing towards the front of the room. Hug your shoulders and release them to keep your arms slightly away from the body, palms facing upward, fingers naturally curled. Pull your shoulders towards your ears and release them. Lift up your right leg to a 30 degrees angle and back. Do the same with your left leg, your right hand and left hand. Spread your legs with your feet hip distance apart and your feet gently tilted on either side. Stretch your heels slightly away from the body. Keep your chin towards the chest, your head straight and not tilted to any side. Face relaxed with a gentle smile and lips gently touching each other, jaws apart. Adjust yourself one last time until you are comfortable and do not move your body till yoga nidra is over.

Body Scanning: Mentally scan your body from top to bottom, right to left, search for any tight or tense areas, consciously release those areas. Be still as still as possible.

Breath Awareness: Take 3 deep yogic breaths. As you breathe in first fill the air into your abdomen, then the chest and then the upper chest and as you exhale first release the air from the upper chest then chest and then the abdomen. Let the breathing be natural now, awareness of breath, awareness of body, contact points of body with the floor....... your natural breath and with every exhalation let go yourself, surrendering body to the floor as one. Feel the sensations inside the body, sensations outside the body, clothes touching the body, air touching the exposed skin.

Sound Awareness: Bring your awareness to the sounds around you. Pick the most distant sound, now pick the next sound, do not analyze it, do not try to find its source or its type, just witness it, pick the sound outside this room/building, jump to the next sound, and to the next. Sounds inside this room, sound within the body, be aware of the inside of the room, walls, ceiling.

Grounding into Yoga Nidra: Feel your body lying on the floor, feel your body, your whole physical body, having awareness of the natural breath, with every breath feel relaxed and tell yourself- "I will keep awake and follow the instructions as I hear them."

Rotation of awareness: Entering into the next stage of yoga nidra you will bring awareness to each part of the body as its name is called out without moving that body part just feel that body part. As the name of that part is called, repeat it in your mind in any language that is comfortable for you, you may even imagine or visualize that body part. Bring your awareness to your right hand thumb, right index finger, middle finger, ring finger, small finger, all five fingers, palm, back of the palm, wrist, forearm, right elbow, right shoulder, the whole right hand, right side of the chest, abdomen, right hip, right thigh, right knee, lower right leg, right ankle, top of the right foot, big toe, 2nd toe, 3rd toe, 4th toe, 5th toe, soul of the right foot, right heel, the whole right foot, the whole right leg, the whole right side of the body, finish with toe.

Moving on to the left hand thumb, left index finger, middle finger, ring finger, small finger, all five fingers, left palm, back of the left palm, left wrist, left forearm, left. elbow, left shoulder, the whole left hand, left side of the chest, abdomen, left hip, left thigh, the left knee, lower leg. left ankle, top of the left foot, big toe, 2nd toe, 3rd toe, 4th toe, 5th toe, soul of the left foot, left heel, the whole left foot, the whole left leg, the whole left side of the body. The whole left side of the body, finishing with the left toe.

Bring your awareness to the back of your body. left and right heels, back of both ankles, both calf muscles, back of both the knees, back of thighs, buttocks, lower back, upper back, shoulder blades, spine, back of left arm , back of right arm, back of the neck, back of the head, the whole back of the body.

Top of the head, forehead, right side of forehead, left side of forehead, right eyebrow, left eyebrow, eyebrow center, right eye, left eye, both eyes together, right ear, left ear, both ears together, right cheeks, left cheeks, both cheeks together, nose, right nostril, left nostril, tip of the nose, upper lip, lower lip, both lips together, tongue, jaw, chin, whole face, throat, chest, abdomen, both hip bones, front of both thighs, both knee caps, front of both lower legs, both the feet, the whole front of the body. Right leg, left leg, both legs together, right hand, left hand, both hands together, trunk, face, head, the whole body, the whole body as one.

Breath Awareness: Bring the awareness to your breath, do not force your breath or change it, keep it natural, just observe your breath, natural ingoing and outgoing breath, passing through the throat, observe the rise and fall of abdomen (pause). Be completely aware of the respiration, maintain awareness and at the same time start counting your breath backwards from 20 as follows: I am inhaling 20, I am exhaling 20, I am inhaling 19, I am exhaling 19, do your own mental counting. Let the breath be natural, total awareness of breathing and counting (pause). In case you miss the count, start again from 20. In case you reach 1 start again from 20.

Externalization: Now relax all the effort and bring your awareness to your breath, movement of the breath, rhythm of the breath, awareness to the rise and fall of chest as you breathe in breathe out, rise and fall of abdomen, feel the sensations in the body, sensations outside the body, your body in this room, inside of this room, walls, ceiling, door, windows, try to locate the position of your body in this room, the color of your clothes, as we finish yoga nidra, bring slight movements into the body. Gently wriggle your fingers, move your toes, move your hands, movements in the leg, shake your head side to side, when you feel you are comfortable turn to the right side on the mat, press the floor with left hand and come to seated position keeping the eyes closed, hands in prayer position, take in three deep breaths and breath out... gently open the eyes. Namaste.

SAMADHI: Samadhi becomes an outcome of asana, pranayama, dhyana and dharana practice. The practitioner is able to do their daily routines with ease, calm, peace and happiness. Yogic lifestyle with yamas and niyamas becomes normal in samadhi.

Specialized Yoga - Restorative Yoga and Yin Yoga

Yoga 'Therapy'

'Therapy' in yoga is not ordinary 'therapy'. It is about some holistic yoga practices that enable the awakening and balancing of life. Yoga 'therapy' is not physiotherapy. Physiotherapy is an offshoot of yoga therapy. In yoga 'therapy', there are no specific tests or diagnosis while modern medical science has techniques like blood test, MRI and so on. Modern science is very good for external diseases which are visible. Yogic techniques can only alleviate the symptoms of invisible diseases like stress, tensions, anxiety, fear, loneliness, depression, inner weaknesses and insomnia. Yoga informs you about imbalances which helps to identify the root causes of ailments or diseases. Yoga 'therapy' involves treatment by changes and corrections of habits or lifestyle. Pantanal says... act according to your limits.

IMPORTANT FACTORS OF YOGA 'THERAPY'
For every case there are 8 points to focus
1. Right lifestyle- There should be a balance between sleep, work and play
2. Right cleaning- Techniques like pranayama, jala neti, shatkarmas, positive thoughts as part of routine life
3. Right posture- The back should not slouch and the right postures can be maintained by correct asanas

4. Right breathing - With correct breathing exercises, you can increase your oxygen intake and capacity and correlate your breath with body and mind

5. Right mindset: A clear and positive mindset as a routine. This can be natural or can be an outcome of good habits, asana and pranayama practice

6. Right diet: Good nutrition food should be had with more protein and balanced carbohydrates. Eat at the same time regularly especially your dinner

7. Right relaxation: Opt for more rest and only peace whenever you are free. For example, you can practice savasana and meditation during your free time.

8. Good sleep: Observe good sleeping habits and if required change your sleeping pattern. Sleep at the same time everyday preferable before 10pm.Try not to sleep for more than 8 hours.

If you are not able to sleep you can practice yoga nidra which is best to connect the gross body and mind in union. You can also opt for savasana with happy and peaceful sankalpas. You can relax your body with yin yoga. Anulom vilom pranayama and bhramari can be practiced before bedtime along with meditation.

After you practice yoga 'therapy' step by step as explained above you can see the results. If you need further help then you can go for natural or ayurvedic or homeopathic medicine

Yoga for obesity

Facts

- Obesity a global problem in today's times
- It is the source of most of the diseases as obesity can lead to any problem in the human body

Symptoms

- Breathlessness
- Lazy feeling
- Feeling the need to sleep more
- Feeling the urge to eat more sometimes
- Lack of interest in physical activity

Causes

- Daily food reach in high calories; eating of high calories food
- Lack of exercise
- Hypertension
- Hypothyroidism
- Genetic causes
- Constipation

Yoga treatment - yoga for slim body and weight loss

- Agnisar kriya 3 - 6 rounds; each round we can do 40-80 movements. For beginners you can practice 2 rounds of 10 counts each
- Trikonasana- 2 times. Breath out and through mouth and hold each round for 11 -21 breaths per minute
- Padahastasana- In the two types of Padahastasana, hold for 10-20 breaths

- Utkatsana - 2 times, for 10 -20 breaths
- Ustrasana - 1 time for 10-20 breaths
- Shashankasana or child pose - for 10-20 breaths
- Chakki chalasana 20 to 50 times in both directions
- Paschimottanasana- 7-10 times for 10 - 15 breaths
- Ardha matsyendrasana- for 11-20 breaths
- Bhujangasana - prone positions are good -3 times - each round for 11- 15 breaths
- Ardha salabhasana - single legs - 3 times - for 10-15 breaths
- Salabhasana - with both legs, 3 times for 10 - 15 breaths
- Dhanurasana - 2 times for 11 - 20 breath
- Naukasana - sitting position- 3 times for 10-20 breaths
- Uttanpadasana- - one leg up - both legs up -3 times for 10 -20 breaths
- Uttan Padangusthasana - 3 times each side for 10 to 20 breaths
- Leg rotation - 5 to 20 times each side
- Yogic cycling - 20 -100 times depend on the capacity
- Pawanmuktasana - 2 to 3 times both sides for 15-20 breaths
- Pranayama -
- Kapalabhatti for 5 -100 times. For beginners you can practice 2 rounds of 10 counts each
- Bhastrika 3 rounds of 15 to 20 breaths. For beginners you can practice 2 rounds of 10 counts each

- Ujjayi 3 rounds of 5 to 10 breaths. For beginners you can practice 2 rounds of 10 counts each
- Bhramari 5 to 15 times
- Shatkarmas- Kunjan kriya, shank prakshalana
- Diet is according to the person's age and current weight. The practitioner can reduce weight with healthy diet

Yoga for Arthritis

The adult human body consists of 206 bones and many joints. The bones provide strength and stability and they also protect our body. The basic structure of bones consists of a soft spiral type of reinforcing protein material surrounded by a black mixture of minerals. This consists mainly of calcium and phosphates.

Bones are a veritable storehouse of mineral materials.

Arthritis is an inflammation of the joints. It can affect one joint or multiple joints. There are more than 100 different types of arthritis with different courses and treatment methods. Two of the most common type are:

Osteoarthritis (OA)
Rheumatoid (RA)

Symptoms
The symptoms of arthritis usually develop over time but they may also appear suddenly. Arthritis is mostly seen in adults over the age of 65 but it can also develop in children, teens and young adults. Arthritis is more common in women than in men.

People who are overweight are more susceptible to arthritis. The most common symptom of arthritis include:

Inflammation of the joints

- Joints pain
- Weaknesses of the bones
- In OA there is pain in the bones of the whole body
- In RA there is redness and acute pain, along with stiffness of the joints and chronic constipation

Causes of arthritis

- Lack of calcium intake through food
- Water and liquid intake is less than required and rising uric acid in the body
- Lack of exercise
- Wrong sleeping habits including sleeping on belly and sleeping on one side with bent knees and bent elbows

Yoga for Arthritis

- Contraction and extension of knees- 50 - 100 times
- Shoulder rotations
- Cat cow pose
- Vakrasana
- Tadasana
- Padahastasana
- Bhujangasana
- Ardha matsyendrasana
- Ardha salabhasana
- Uttanpadasana
- Pawanmuktasana
- Setu Bandhasana

- Bhramari pranayama
- Brahma mudra
- Bhastrika pranayama
- Kapalabhatti - 50- 100 reps
- Anulom vilom
- Savasana

Exercises for hand

- Fingers on shoulders - bend and straighten hands forward - 10 - 20 times slowly -
- Fingers on shoulders bend and straighten hands sideways - 10 - 20 times slowly
- Static full arm rotations - 10-20 times
- Fingers on shoulders - shoulder rotations- 10 times both directions
- Fingers on shoulders - touch shoulders, open elbows sideways and bring the elbows back together
- Fingers on shoulders; open elbows bring the elbows down - 10 - 20 times
- Full arm rotations - 10 times in both directions, slowly with awareness and continuous breathing

Exercises for wrists

- Wrists up and down
- Wrists sideways and back with fingers open
- Wrist rotations and opposite side wrist rotations, with open and closed fingers
- Fingers together and open apart slowly with awareness and continuous breathing
- Hold one hand up for a minimum of 1 minute with eyes closed and feel the pose and then

slowly bring down the hand. Do this on both sides
- You can lift both hands up also
- You can stand or sit in to a chair and perform these wrist exercises

Exercises for the hands

- Hands - sideways and back
- Hands front and back
- Hands up and down
- Upper fingers - bend and straighten 10 - 20 times
- All the fingers - open and close with thumb in and thumb out alternatively
- Keep the fingers straight and bend fingers in both directions
- Pull each finger - 10 times, relax with deep breathing and normal breathing
- Fingerlock and move hands front and back
- Fingerlock and move hand up and down
- Fingerlock and rotate wrists, change the fingerlock direction
- Put thumb inside and make fist, keep awareness with the breath
- Hands on floor, lift up fingers one by one with the other hand
- Fingerlock and press and open upper fingers
- Fingerlock and take both hands up and breathe normally for 6 to 15 times

Exercises for the feet

The same thing as is done for the feet, sitting on chair or floor or in the standing position

- Hold toes up and down for the count of 6 for one leg at a time and for both legs - 10 times
- Sit in ardha padmasana, then hold and pull toes
- Foot massage with thumbs
- Flex toes - 10 to 50 times
- Point toes and flex feet - 10 to 50 times
- Tadasana- stand on heels and toes - 10 times
- Ankle rotations in standing and/or sitting position - 10 to 50 times
- Press toes in the mat/floor in the standing position
- Press on sides of feet in the standing position
- Bend and hug knees in the standing position - 10 times
- Press kneecaps up and release - 5 to 50 times
- Contract kneecaps and release in the sitting position - 5 to 50 times

Exercises in the sitting and lying positions

- Lags a little apart keep hands by side of the hips, move and rotate legs and touch toes together and then toes apart - 10 - 15 times
- Ankle rotations slowly in both directions
- Press toes to the mat/ floor by raising heels
- One hand up and down, slowly - 5 to 20 times
- Both hands up and down, slowly - 5 to 20 times
- Bend your knee and keep the ankle over the opposite thigh (as in ardha baddha) and hold

your foot. Rotate the ankle for some time. Do the same in the other side by changing the leg position

- Hands to side, bend and straighten legs - 5 to 20 times
- Drop elbows, bend and straighten knees - 5 to 20 times
- Lying down, move one leg up and down at a time - 5 to 10 times
- Lying down, move both legs up and down - 5 to 10 times
- Lying down, bend and straighten one knee at a time - 5 to 10 times
- Lying down, bend and straighten both knees at a time - 5 to 10 times
- Lying down, bend knees, touch hands to knees and rotate the knees in both directions
- Lying down, bend knees and lift one leg up and down at a time - 5 to 10 times
- Lying down, bend knees and lift both leg up and down - 5 to 10 times
- Lying down-, hand by side open the knees outwards and close the knees inwards
- Sit in Gomukhasana and clap your feet with your hands. Change the feet position and repeat
- Clap hands for 5 to 50 times in the sitting or lying down position
- This is a specialized class and add gentle breathing exercises like yogic breathing, anulom vilom pranayama and bhramari pranayama

Yoga for Heart Problems

- The human heart is a marvelous organ. Due to modernization, lots of problems are faced by the heart. Hence one should know yoga therapy for various heart problems
- The heart function is to circulate blood through all parts of the body. The heart never stops even for a moment in its activities during its lifetime.
- Although the heart is a single organ, it actually consists of two pumps. It receives blood from all parts of the body and propels it to the lungs. There the blood drops its load of carbon dioxide and receives a fresh supply of oxygen. The oxygenated blood then passes to the left side of the heart and from there it is pumped again to all parts of the body
- One of the most common complications of heart disease is heart failure. Heart failure occurs when your heart cannot pump enough blood to meet your body needs. Heart failure can result from many forms of heart disease.

Symptoms

- Chest pain
- Left arm pain
- Breathless while resting
- Headache
- Temporary impotence
- ECG positive
- Abnormally early heart beats
- High blood pressure
- Fainting
- Dizziness

Causes

- Wrong eating habits
- Obesity
- High blood cholesterol
- Lack of regular exercise
- Stress
- Anxiety
- Swelling of body
- Blood pressure on heart due to gas and constipation

Yoga Therapy

- Shashankasana - 2 minutes
- Vakrasana - 1 time
- Kandharasana - (bridge pose lift your hip up) 10 - 11 rounds
- Bhujangasana- 2-3 times
- Ardha halasana plough pose - 2 times
- Uttanpadasana-- lying down with your back legs up - 2-3 times
- Brahma mudra
- Agnisar kriya - 5 times
- Udiyana bandha - 3 rounds
- Anulom vilom - 11 - 21 times
- Ujjayi pranayama 11- 21 rounds
- Bhramari pranayama- 10-11 times
- Savasana - 5-7 minutes
- These asanas will make your heart stronger

Yoga for Women's Problems

- Women's problems almost entirely arise from imbalances in female hormones. These important hormones are produced in two pairs of almond shaped organs known as ovaries. They are deep in the pelvis one on each side of the uterus or womb

There are 2 major female hormones
- Estrogen
- Progesterone
- Estrogen gives enormous drive energy and stamina. Progesterone has a special function of its own. Any Imbalance in these hormones causes symptoms like:

Back ache
Painful menstruation
Chronic constipation
Vaginal discharge
Sleeplessness
Hunger
Premenstrual tension
Heavy bleeding
Pain in lower abdomen
Obesity
Lumbar spondylitis
Low blood pressure
Irritability
Early menopause

Causes
- Sleeping in the belly
- Always sleeping on left side
- Long hours in bed
- Fibroids
- Hypotension

- Bending left leg while sleeping
- Stiff back
- Lack of exercise
- Hypothyroidism

Yoga for Women's Problems
- Brahma mudra
- Tadasana 5 repetitions for 5 breaths each
- Kati chakrasana in both directions with normal breathing
- Vajrasana 2 - 3 repetitions for 10 breaths each
- Janu sirshasana 2 - 3 repetitions for 10 breaths each
- Paschimottanasana 2 - 3 repetitions for 10 breaths each
- Shashankasana 2 - 3 repetitions for 10 breaths each
- Vakrasana 2 - 3 repetitions for 10 breaths each
- Some simple basic side stretches in Baddhakonasa
- Open legs sideways
- Cat cow 5 to 25 repetitions with continuous breathing
- Trikonasana 2 - 3 repetitions for 10 breaths each
- Padahastasana 2 - 3 repetitions for 10 breaths each
- Bhujangasana 2 - 3 repetitions for 10 breaths each
- Ardha salabhasana - raise one leg up at a time 3 to 6 repetitions with focus on the breath
- Dhanurasana 2 repetitions for 10 breaths each
- Pawanmuktasana 2 to 3 repetitions

- Setu Bandhasana 2 to 3 repetitions
- Brahma mudra with normal breathing for 1 - 15 minutes
- Anulom vilom -10 rounds
- Bhramari -10 rounds
- Meditation for 5 to 25 minutes
- Savasana / Deep relaxation technique/ yoga nidra - 5 to 15 minutes

Yoga for back pain and slipped disc and lumbar spondylitis

Symptoms

- Pain in the lower back mainly center part
- Pain in both or one calf muscles
- Heel ache or pain
- Burning or lack of control on urination
- Difficulties in long hours standing, walking and climbing
- Lack of balancing

Causes

- Sitting position for a long time
- Wrong sleeping habits
- Sleeping on one side - addictive pose
- Loose bed
- Aging
- Lack of exercise and muscle power
- Continuous forward bending
- Heavy weight lifting
- Wrong pose due to wrong asana practice wrong alignment instructions

Contraindications of back pain

- While having back pain we should avoid forward bending
- If bending forward then don't push too much only bend a little bit
- If bending forward bend knees while bending down
- Don't do forward bending, heavy weight lifting
- Do the recommended asanas

Asanas

- Tadasana with heels up - 5 rounds
- Trikonasana - 5 rounds
- Hasta padasana -   slowly 5 times with awareness
- Cat - cow - marjariasana - 7-8 times
- Kati chakrasana for the spinal twist- 5 rounds
- Shashankasana child pose -.any variation for 2 minutes
- Bhujangasana- sphinx- hold face - straight hand
- Ardha salabhasana- single leg salabhasana 3- 4 times
- Eka pada uttanasana - one leg up at a time
- Bend your leg and hug your knee in the standing position - 5 times
- Dhanurasana (if back pain is less)
- Downward facing dog (if back pain is less)
- Single leg Pawanmuktasana
- Pawanmuktasana- 5.times
- Setu Bandhasana- hands by side of waist or fingerlock - 5 or 6 times
- Put pillow under your back and just relax
- Drop knees sideways
- Vipatikarani
- Savasana- 5 minutes

- Anulom vilom - om meditation

Depression, insomnia and anxiety

- Depression is combined with feelings of sadness, irritability and anxiety. The inability to sleep or disturbed sleep are a few of the symptoms of depression

Symptoms
- Lack of interest is any kind of work
- Difficulties in sleeping
- Feeling of tension
- Phobias

Causes of depression
- Anxiety and insomnia
- Hormone imbalance in brain due to stress
- Lack of circulation in brain
- Wrong posture of sleeping
- Using big pillows
- Watching TV in the bed
- Sleeping on belly for whole night
- Working on table for long hours
- Low BP

Yoga Therapy
- Shashankasana
- Cat
- Ustrasana
- Padahastasana
- Padangusthasana
- Trikonasana
- Bhujapidasana
- Dhanurasana

- Uttanpadasana
- Viparita Karani
- Anulom vilom
- Bhramari
- Savasana
- Meditation
- Jal neti sutra neti

TRATAKA

- 'Trataka' is steady gazing at a particular point or object without winking. Though this is one of the six purification exercises, it is mainly intended for developing concentration and mental focusing. It is very useful for yoga practitioners as it can be included within their regular practice. This is an effective method for the control of the mind and one can depend on the results of this practice.
- Tips for the practitioners for the Candle Flame Gazing Technique or Jyoti Trataka:
- Trataka must be practiced on a steady flame. The candle or the diya should be 3 to 4 feet or 1 meter in front of you on a height such that the flame is at eye level
- Trataka can be performed in darkness during the night or in a semi dark room during the day time. Try to avoid a bright room
- Try and eliminate drafts by closing the windows so that the flame can be steady
- Find a peaceful place and keep your candle or diya ready
- Remove your glasses, wrist watches, belts and be comfortable
- Sit with your head, neck, and spine upright
- During the entire practice, always open your eyes with a few blinks

- When you open your eyes, don't look at the flame right away. Start looking at the floor and then slowly bring your gaze onto the flame
- During trataka practices, try not to blink or move the eyeballs
- During palming, don't let the palms touch or press the eyeballs. Palms, not the fingers, cover the eyes. Do palming very slowly and with deep breathing and awareness. The palms are placed in such a way that there is complete darkness to the eyes
- The facial muscles, eyebrows, and eyelids should remain totally relaxed with a beautiful smile on your face. During the practice, the practitioner should always avoid any kind of strain to the eyes
- Trataka should be performed after asanas and pranayamas practice

Jyoti Trataka routine with a duration of about 30 min.

1. . Starting prayer (OM Sahana Vavatu.....)
2. We can start trataka with eye exercises to reduce the strain on the eye muscles during the practice:
3. Note: During any eye exercise, you must not move your head. Only eyeballs move. Keep the gaze closer to you and not far away from you whilst performing eye exercises

a) Up and down or vertical movements of the eyeballs: Number of rounds: 10. Palming: simple palming

b) Right and left or horizontal movement of the eyeballs: Number of rounds: 10. Palming: simple palming

c) Diagonal movement of eyeballs: Right up and left down, Left up and right down, 10 rounds of each is to be performed followed by press and release palming

d) Rotational or circular movement of eyeballs: Clockwise, Anti-clockwise, 10 rounds of each followed by palming with constant pressure

4. Candle flame gazing (at 3 stages)

a) The first step: Focusing on the whole flame

Start looking at the floor and then slowly bring your gaze into the flame. Bring your focus onto the whole flame and continuously gaze at the flame. There should be no blinking or winking. The gaze should be smooth and effortless. Use your will power and ignore watering or irritation in the eyes. Gaze for 30 – 60 sec. After that do press and release palming.

b) The second step: Intensive focusing on the tip of the wick

Open your eyes with a few blinks. Start looking at the floor and then slowly bring your gaze up onto the tip of the flame. Bring your focus onto the tip of the flame and continuously gaze at it. There should be no blinking or winking. The gaze should be smooth and effortless. Use your will power and ignore watering or irritation in the eyes. Gaze for 30 – 60 sec. After that do palming with constant pressure

c) The third step: De-focusing

Open your eyes with a few blinks. Start looking at the floor and then slowly bring your gaze up onto the whole flame for a few seconds. Slowly defocus your attention, inhale and exhale and have a de-focused look at the flame. Keep expanding your vision. Slowly see the aura around the flame, gradually becoming bigger and bigger. Slowly also see the small-small light particles around the flame. Enjoy this expansive state for about a minute

Now, again bring back your focus on the whole flame for a few seconds. Close your eyes and visualize the "after-image" of the flame between your eyebrows. As the image disappears, go for simple palming with Bhramari (5 rounds)

1. Silence: At the end, with eyes closed, sit quietly for some time.
2. Closing prayer (Asato ma sadgamaya....)

Benefits of trataka:

Physical:

1. Helps with reducing and removing eye strain by improving the
stamina of muscles and deep relaxation to them.
2. It makes eyes clear, bright, and radiant.
3. It cleanses the tear glands and purifies the optical system.

Therapeutic:

1. Observatory refraction errors get corrected as the external eye
muscles improve
2. Strengthens the ciliary muscles (short and long sightedness are
benefited)
3. Balances the nervous system relieving nervous tension, anxiety,
depression, and insomnia
4. Those who suffer from insomnia and mental tension should perform

this practice of gazing continuously or 10-15 minutes before going
to sleep at night

Spiritual:
1. Helps to develop concentration and improves memory
2. Helps to develop a strong willpower
3. It is an excellent preparation for meditation

Limitations and contraindications:
1. Glaucoma patients should avoid or do under proper guidance.
2. Epileptics should avoid candle flame gazing. They can, however
choose a totally steady object to gaze on
3. People with eye infection should avoid it
4. In case of burning sensation in the eyes or headache, one should
avoid this practice

General benefits:
Through the practice of trataka:
1. Diseases of the eyes are removed.
2. Eyesight improves.
3. Many have thrown away their spectacles after taking to this practice.
4. Willpower is developed.
5. Vikshepa (sorrow) is destroyed.
6. Steadies the mind.
7. Clairvoyance, thought reading, psychic cure and other Siddhis are obtained very easily.

Similar Practices:

- Keep the picture of Lord Krishna, Rama, Narayana, Devi or any Lord in front of you. Look at it steadily without winking. Gaze at the head; then at the body; then at the legs. Repeat the same process again and again. When your mind calms down, look at a particular place only. Be steady till tears begin to flow. Then close the eyes and mentally visualize the picture.
- Gaze on a black dot on a white wall or draw a black mark on a piece of white paper and hang it on the wall in front of you. Practice trataka with it
- Draw the picture OM on a piece of paper and have it before your seat. Do trataka on it
- Lie down on an open terrace and gaze at a particular bright star or on the full moon. After some time, you will see different colors of lights. Again some time later, you will see only a particular star throughout, and all other surrounding stars will disappear. When you gaze at the moon, you will see only a bright moon on a black background. At times you will see a huge mass of light all around you. When gazing becomes more intense, you can also see two or three moons of the same size and at times you cannot see any moon at all even though your eyes may be wide open.
- Select at random any place in the open sky in the morning or evening hours and gaze at it steadily and do trataka
- Look at a mirror and gaze at the pupil of your eye
- Some people do trataka at the space between the two eyebrows or at the tip of the nose.

Even while walking, one can do trataka at the tip of the nose

- Advanced students can do trataka at the inner Chakras (Padmas). The Muladhara, Anahata, Ajna and Sahasrara are the important centers for trataka practice
- Keep a ghee-lamp before you and gaze at the flames. Some astral entities give Darshan through the flames.
- Very few Yogis do trataka on the sun. It requires the help of an experienced person by their side. They begin by gazing on the rising sun and after gradual practice they do trataka on the sun even in the midday. They get some special Siddhis (psychic powers) by this practice. All are not fit for this Sun Trataka Sadhana. The Guru will prescribe some oil to rub on your head to avoid such serious troubles and to cool the system. You should apply honey to your eyes at night when you practice sun gazing

All the first 9 exercises will suit everyone and they are harmless. The last one, sun-gazing should not be attempted until you get the help of an experienced person / teacher.

More instructions:

When you do the Trataka in your meditation room, sit in your favorite asana (posture), Siddhasana or Padmasana. At other times you can do it in a standing or sitting posture. Trataka can be done even while walking. As you walk along the streets, do not look hither and thither. Gaze at the tip of the nose or toes. Therefore, no particular asana is required for this Sadhana

When you gaze at a picture, it is trataka. When you close your eyes and mentally visualize the picture, it is Saguna Dhyana (meditation with form). When you associate the attributes of God such as omnipresence, omnipotence, omniscience, purity, perfection; the name and the form of the object of trataka will automatically disappear and you will enter into Nirguna Dhyana (abstract meditation)

Do trataka for two minutes to start with. Then gradually and carefully increase the period. Do not be impatient. Gradual steady practice is required. Then you will advance in this practice and will be able to do trataka for a longer duration

Those who cannot gaze steadily for a second in spite of several attempts need not worry much. They can close their eyes and gaze at an imaginary spot at the space between the two eyebrows.

Those who have very weak eyes can do trataka after closing their eyes and focusing on any imaginary spot within. Do not tax your eyes by over-practicing

When you feel tired, close your eyes and keep your mind on the object of trataka

Do this for one month regularly to experience the full benefits.

Do not shake the body when you sit and do trataka

Trataka improves eyesight. Many who have had some eye troubles have realized immense benefits by trataka. It prepares the mind undoubtedly for perfect Dhyana and Samadhi. The same object of gazing will appear as something else during the practice. You will have many other visions. Different people have different experiences. You will not even believe certain things when others tell you of their experiences.

The Teaching Methodology

- The sequence flow should be connected
- Start the class with warm up exercises
- The sequence flow should be connected
- Start the class - take a sequence - eg:
- open leg sequence
- Try to remember what you can do in the next pose
- You can make your own sequences

Other popular classifications or themes in a yoga class

1. Hip Opening Pose: Baddhakonasa - Open legs sideways - variations
2. Forward bending
3. Back bending
4. Hamstrings
5. Quadriceps
6. Weight loss
7. Power yoga
8. Flexibility yoga
9. Ashtanga sequence
10. Yin yoga
11. Kundalini yoga
12. Chakra yoga

Joint Movement Exercises
Warm up exercises
- Take a sequence - For example: In the sitting posture; open leg sideways sequence
- Take gentle sun salutations
- Take the standing poses sequences

- Tadasana - variations
- Ardhakati - variations
- Band bend - bend forward
- Sun salutations and modifications
- Ashtanga poses
- Balancing asanas

- Lying down with the back poses

- Lying down with the chest poses

- Hip Opening poses: for example: Baddhakonasa and opening legs sideways **with** variations

- More standing asanas

- More sitting asanas

- Lying asanas in the Spine and Prone positions

- Twisting asanas

- Inversion asanas

- Balancing asanas - maybe on one hand one leg on the hip on the arms

- Meditation asanas

- Forward bending poses

- Backward bending poses - also in the sitting , standing and lying down positions

- Padmasana group asanas

To create flow, you can mix all these asanas and make the class. Try to remember what you can do in the next pose. You can make your own sequences.

SEQUENCING PRINCIPALS

Creating a sequence is an art and is crucial for the success of the yoga class.

What is sequencing

Sequencing is to build a complete and effective yoga class that enables the transition from one pose to another comfortably and easily. Sequencing a class requires a yoga teacher to assess and anticipate the needs and capabilities of the whole class. The class should enable ease and effective balance and stability.

The movement into poses and into the next pose has a connection. The simplest sequence is called a 'vinyasa' where the body, mind and breath are consciously synchronized by using adequate transitional movement between poses. For example, in sun salutation when we start with 'tadasana' or mountain pose with both hands by the side, we move into 'urdhva hastasana' which means 'both hands up' with an inhale and then continue towards the back bend and forward bend. The movement and breathing are correlated and enable the practitioner to have greater awareness, steadiness and ease. When the practitioner is not able to focus on breath and movement synchrony, it is a sign to slow down or decrease the intensity of the practice.

Why do you need sequencing?

Though there is no definite sequence that is best or most effective, sequences that make sense depend on the number of students, the capacity and the different abilities of the practitioners. In this manner, the sequences are made to be safe, healthy and appropriate to the practitioners. The yoga teacher should integrate their knowledge about asanas, pranayama, yoga anatomy and philosophy. They should be creative and can use the resources like templates and the teachings of other yoga teachers, but should be made appropriate to address the needs of movement and flexibility. In this manner, the teacher should be able to flexibly create sequences integrating body, mind and spirit and move the practitioners into a deeper practice.

Characteristics of a good sequence
The sequence should be made with correct information and knowledge about the element or theme that you are teaching'
It should be beautiful and create a deeply satisfying practice. At the same time, it should effectively meet the intention and objective of the practitioner and the class.
The sequence should efficiently guide the students in a simple manner into an integrated, safe and deeper yoga practice.

Different ways of sequencing: Yoga Themes
Sequencing can be based on themes that the yoga teacher makes for the needs of the practitioners.
Sequencing is done
- Towards an advanced pose
- Therapeutic or restorative
- A spiritual theme like bhakti or kundalini, yama, niyamas, gratefulness, mindfulness, inspiring quote
- Yoga for stress relief
- Yoga for beginners
- Yoga for twisting

- Yoga for the core
- Yoga for the hips, thighs, upper back, lower back
- Yoga for a slim body, love handles
- Power and weight loss yoga
- Yoga with chair
- Yoga with ball
- Yoga with stick

The teacher may take a notebook and make a note of some questions that they might ask themselves about the sequence and the yoga class:

1. Time of the yoga class - morning or evening
2. Season and months of the class, the phases of the moon that determine the energy level. A yin or restorative class is to be practiced during new moon and full moon days
3. Festivals and world sports events and other world events
4. The length of the class
5. New knowledge. feelings and experience of students in the class
6. What would serve the students best and what they would enjoy

Create some sample sequences. Creating a yoga sequence is an art and is crucial for the success of the yoga class.

HOW TO SEQUENCE THE CLASS

- Start in sitting standing or in vajrasana
- Greeting relaxation om chanting 5 mins
- Warm up - 5-7 min , same for standing postures to warm up
- Lying down with the back
- Inversions - Sarvangasana and head stand
- Lying down with the chest
- Kneeling positions and gate positions with variations
- Sitting positions
- Pranayama and Savasana

1) Sitting down with the legs front

- Different types of positions- 5 poses on each side – you can make a sequence

- You have to check what the next pose you can do and you need to remember also what pose you can make

- Paschimottanasana - twisting

- Baddhakonasa - poses

- Until now, you can prepare this one class for nearly 20 - 25 minutes

Next is

2) Lying down with the back

3) Or standing on knees - sideways bending; back bending

3) Gate pose open hands shoulder level sideways bending - bend forward – twisting - needle the thread single hand back bend

For all these positions, you can do
- Simple
- Intermediate
- Advanced

6) Next comes cat and cow pose which requires core strength - Check the position – take low lunge and back bend- low lunge all the positions- then take pigeon pose all the positions

7) Downward facing dog positions

- Warrior
- Back bending
- Forward bending
- Twisting

HOW TO SEQUENCE THE CLASS - Teaching Methodology

1) Starting

- Start in sitting standing or in vajrasana

- Greeting relaxation om chanting, some pranayama 8 mins

- Warm up for 5-7 minutes, same is for standing and sitting positions. These consist of
  - Head rotation
  - Wrist rotation
  - Shoulder rotation
  - Arm rotation
  - Twisting
  - Sideway bending
  - Bending back
  - Bending forward
  - Hip rotation and movements
  - Knee movements and rotation
  - Cardiovascular poses like yogic marching and squatting

2) Next Step

- With different types of stances, make a sequence with 2 or more poses on each side
- You can also opt for single asanas done on both sides
- You have to check what the next pose can be done and you need to remember also what

pose you can make that can form a comfortable and effective sequence

Stance 1: Sitting Position

Both the legs front position
-   Paschimottanasana can be done with forward fold
-   Twisting, side bending and back bending
-   Naukasana
-

Baddha Konasana position
-   Bring both the feet together and swing the knees together
-   Press the knees down with the palms
-   Bend forward
-   Bend back
-   Twisting

Until now this will take nearly 20 - 25 minutes. The next 30 minutes can be constructed by choosing from the other 9 stances which I have made. The choice of asanas will depend on the objective of the class. For example: back bending, forward bending, hip opening, strong and flexible legs, weight loss, restorative, specific illnesses or injuries and so on.

The other asanas in the sitting position are:
- Both legs straight waist distance apart
- One leg straight and the other leg knees bent 90 degrees
- Janu sirshasana
- Ardha baddha paschimmotanasana
- Ardha mukho paschimmotanasana
- Ardha matsyendrasana
- Marchenasana

- Ardha paschimottanasana
- Purvatasana
- Reverse table pose
- Bakasana
- Titibasana
- Malasana
- Vajrasana
- Animal pose
- Gomukhasana
- Vakrasana
- Padmasana
- Naukasana
- Kumar asana
- Wide legged forward folds and variations
- Single led outwards forward folds and variations

Each of these stances can have variations:
- Forward bend,
- Back bend,
- Side bending
- Twisting

The hands in any and all of these stances could be
- Both hands opened sideways at shoulder level
- Both hands up
- Both hands forward
- Palms down or elbows down on the floor
- In prayer position
- In reverse prayer position
- Elbow locked behind the back
- Elbow locked above the head
- In cactus position

- In gomukhasana position
- Both hands behind the head
- Both hands or one hand on the waist
- Both hands or one hand straight by side
- Fingers in fist position

Stance 2:
Lying down with the back: There are many poses in this position including yogic cycling, yogic leg rotation, yogic leg lifts, yogic crunches, setu bandhasana, sarvangasana, yogic leg drops sideways, supta padangusthasana, supta eka pada kapotasana, sideways twisting, stretching, hamstring stretches, pavanmuktasana, rolling and, chakrasana. You can make a sequence designed to fit within your schedule and the theme of the class.

Stance 3:
Standing on knees - there are many poses that can be customized in this position including sideways bending with variations in the hand positions; kapotasana, supta baddha virasan, back bending, ustrasana, single hand backbending continuously,

Stance 4:
Gate pose: Opening hands shoulder level or both arms up, you can choose sideways bending, bending forward, extended triangle, warrior 1 and 2 pattern,, drop elbow down other hand up which is like needle the thread, single hand back bend, and both arms down skandasana.

In this manner depending on the variations that you choose, for all these positions, you can do practice at these levels:

- Simple
- Intermediate
- Advanced

Stance 5:
Lying down with the chest positions : child pose bhujangasana, bhujangasana twisting, Dhanurasana with variations, sphinx, upward facing dog, superman variations, locust variations or salabhasana single leg and both legs together

Stance 6:
Cat and cow pose
- Spinal stretch
- Single hand single leg
- Hold the leg
- Chest down
- Needle the thread
- Single leg - tiger - leg lifts and crunches - half plank
- Tiger core - bend and straighten knee sideways

Stance 7:
Downward facing dog: This position can be practiced by itself or it can be used for transitions into other poses by changing the stance or into a vinyasa leading to
- Ardha chandrasana
- Ardha chakrasana
- Wild thing
- Handstand
- Lizard
- Eka pada kapotasana
- Plank and plank variations

- Bird of paradise

Stance 8:
Standing Positions with all the variations:
- Tadasana
- Purvatasana
- All warrior positions
- Parsvakonasana and reverse extended triangle
- Parvatattanasan
- Trikonasana and reverse triangle
- Vrikshasana
- Utthita baddha paschimmotanasana
- Standing gomukhasana
- Utthita padangusthasana
- Hastasana, Back bending
- Forward bending, pada hastasana
- Twisting all variations
- Standing split
- Tadasana with variations
- Ardhakati chakrasana with variations
- Uttanasana twisting
- Prasarita padottanasana all variations
- Utkatsana with variations

Stance 9:
- Low lunge with variations; hanumanasana

Stance 10:
Inversions: the positions in which the heart is above the head is called as downward dog, inversions, Extended puppy pose, legs up the wall pose, shoulder stand, plow pose, dolphin pose, head stand, handstand, tripod or forearm stand or salamba sirshasana , feathered peacock pose

Sequencing - Power, Weight Loss, Vinyasa

Sun Salutation

Traditional surya namaskar and variations
Surya Namaskar a and b and variations

Sun salutation, which signifies prayer and respect for the sun, is also called surya namaskar and consists of a flow of asanas.

- Traditional yoga has a set of 12 asanas and is known as traditional surya namaskar.

- Ashtanga yoga has two types of yoga which are Surya Namaskar A and Surya Namaskar B

Sequencing and alignment for traditional surya namaskar _ a complete hatha yoga practice in itself addressing different parts of the body

- Traditional surya namaskar is composed of 12 classical yoga poses which are practiced with the flow of breath
- It is practiced on each side of the body
- The benefits includes stretching and strengthening of the body

The 12 steps of surya namaskar are:

1. Pranamasana (Prayer pose)

2. Hasta Uttanasana (Raised arms pose)

3. Hastapadasana (Standing forward bend)

4. Ashwa Sanchalanasana (Equestrian pose)

5. Dandasana (Stick pose)

6. Ashtanga Namaskar (Salute with eight parts)

7. Bhujangasana (Cobra pose)

8. Adho Mukha Svanasana (Downward facing dog pose)

9. Ashwa Sanchalanasana (Equestrian pose)

10. Hastapadasana (Standing forward bend)

11. Hasta Uttanasana (Raised arms pose)

12. Tadasana (Mountain Pose)

TRADITIONAL SURYA NAMASKAR DEFINITIONS AND ALIGNMENTS

1. Pranamasana (Prayer pose)

A centering asana	A transitional pose	Performed in the standing, sitting or squatting position
In traditional surya namaskar, it is performed in the standing position	The palms are pressed in front of the heart center with the palms facing up	The shoulders are rolled down the back
The elbows are rested towards the side of the ribcage with normal breathing	It is generally the first and last asana of any yoga session	It is an easy and effortless posture
Strengthens the nervous system and improves digestion	It maintains body posture	Improves mental calmness

2. Hasta Uttanasana (Raised arms pose)

Stand straight and breathe normally. Keep your feet together and body straight	2. Now raise your hands (to salute the sun) above your head while breathing in deeply.	3. Now bend your trunk and head a little backward to create a slight curve at the same time as you raise your arms
4. Hold this	This pose	This pose

Stand straight and breathe normally. Keep your feet together and body straight	2. Now raise your hands (to salute the sun) above your head while breathing in deeply.	3. Now bend your trunk and head a little backward to create a slight curve at the same time as you raise your arms
pose for 10-15 seconds.	expands the chest and rib cage and helps in full entail of oxygen	lengthens the front part of the body and strengthens the back muscles
This pose helps strengthen the shoulder neck chest and abdomen muscles	Increases flexibility and mobility and helps increase height	Primary movement: Flexion in both the hips and extension in the spine

3. Hastapadasana (Standing forward bend)

Stand straight with your feet together and hands by your side	2. Inhale raise both your hands up	3. Exhale, bend forward, touch your toes and hold your ankles
Try to keep your knees straight and touch your forehead to the knee	Stay in this position for 6 second while suspending the breath for 6 seconds	This pose may be held for no longer than 2 minutes while breathing normally

Inhale raise your arms up and exhale bring your hands down to the side	Contraindications: Hypertension, cardiac ailments, pregnancy, peptic ulcers, hernia, cervical spondylitis , slipped disk	This pose is beneficial for the back, hip and hamstring muscles
Clams your nervous system	Gently massages your abdominal muscles	Primary movements: Flexion of the hips and extension of the spine

4. Ashwa Sanchalanasana (Equestrian pose)

The 4th and 9th pose in traditional sun salutation	In surya namaskar, Padahastasana is the starting position for the pose	Inhale, take the left leg behind while bending the right knee without changing its position and by keeping the knee in line with the ankle
While stretching the left leg backwards, keep the hand straight while touching the floor.	Arch the back and tilt the head slightly backwards. Look straight ahead	It tones the abdominal muscles, gives flexibility to the leg muscles and enables equilibrium and balance in the

		body. It prepares the body for deeper backbends.
The pose may be entered through Tadasana, Padahastasana or through adho mukha svanasana	Contraindications: Avoid this pose if you have any type of knee injury, look down in case of neck pain, late pregnancies	The spiritual awareness is on the ajna and the Muladhara chakra

5. Dandasana: Stick Pose

It is a seated pose and is also known as the staff pose. It is a restorative pose and affects the spleen and stomach meridians.	It is a foundation pose for all seated poses and also a transition pose	It strengthens hips, pelvis and lower back, lengthens lower back and help open the chest
Sit with legs straight and back straight and hand next to the hips. Lengthen your spine and press your hands to the ground	Bend you elbows or come to your fingertips to adjust the proportion between the arms and torso	Keep the feet engaged, the legs active and the core engaged.
Keep the shoulders away	The shoulders stacked over the	The spiritual awareness is on

from the ears. Keep the spine straight. The neck should be in line with the spine.	hips with strong arms and hands. Do not tilt the pelvis backward or put weight on the wrists	the Manipura Chakra (solar plexus), Sacral Chakra (swadisthan chakra) and the Root Chakra (Muladhara chakra)

6. Ashtanga Namaskara (salute with eight parts)

In Sanskrit, ashta means eight, anga means part and namaskara means salutation	The body is in contact with the floor in eight locations during the pose as a mark of respect. In the prone position, you **touch the ground with your feet, knees, palms, chest, and chin**.	From the downward facing dog or from the cat pose or from the plank pose, gently drop your knees to the floor and tuck your toes, Now bring your chest to the floor, then finally bring your forehead/chin to the floor. Keep breathing smoothly throughout the pose
- The elbows should be closer to the chest - The shoulders are in between the palms and	The anatomy of this pose are the biceps, feet soles, wrist, the quadriceps and the hip flexors	Contraindications: this pose should not be practiced if the practitioner - Has carpal

are rolled up forward so that the chest can expand - The hips are raised and the belly is engaged so that the chin or forehead touches the floor - Maintain this position as you are comfortable with slow breathing - raise your chin, chest, shoulders and let go of the belly and knees to move to the next pose	The variations include: 1. One legged four limbed staff pose where one leg is lifted up 2. Four limbed staff pose where the head and chest are lifted up	tunnel syndrome - Women in pregnancy after the first trimester - After any kind of surgery especially an abdominal surgery - Has neck, wrist or shoulder injury
Follow Up Poses - Bhujangasana (Cobra Pose) - Urdhva Mukha Svanasana (Upward-Facing Dog Pose) - Balasana (Child Pose) - Cat pose - Adho Mukha	The benefits of this asana: - Massages internal organs - Makes the spine strong and flexible - Regulates the endocrine system - Strengthens the upper body	The spiritual awareness is on the: Mooladhara (Root) Chakra, Manipura (Solar Plexus) Chakra, and Swadhisthana (Sacral) Chakra

Svanasana (Downward Facing Dog Pose)		

7. Bhujangasana (Cobra pose)

This is done lying down on the belly and is an energizing backbend pose	You'll be coming into cobra from ashtanga namaskara or by simply lying down on your belly	- Place your palms on the ground directly under your shoulders - Keep your elbows closer to your body - Pause for a moment looking straight ahead, keeping your neck in neutral position and anchoring your hips to the floor - Inhale and lift your chest off the floor keeping the elbows closer. Keep your low ribs to the floor and your elbow closer - Your neck should be in the neutral position and not lifted

		up. Your gaze should be on the mat - Exhale and release back to the floor
Follow up poses: - Downward facing dog or adho mukha svanasana - Cat pose - Child pose	The variations to this pose include - Sphinx - Urdhva mukha svanasana or Upward facing dog pose - Hands free cobra - Baby cobra or ardha bhujangasana	- Increases mobility of the spine - strengthens spinal support muscles - Helps relieve back pain - Can alleviate the over hunched back that has resulted from too much sitting
To reduce the strain on the back: - Increase the bend in the elbows or - Walk the hands further forward	Contraindications: Do not do bhujangasana if you have - Carpal tunnel syndrome - injury to back arm or shoulders - If you recently had an abdominal surgery - If you are pregnant	The spiritual awareness is on the anahata or the heart chakra

8. Adho Mukha Svanasana (Downward facing dog pose)

It is a pose in - Sun salutation - Or done many times in a yoga class especially in a vinyasa class - It is also the first pose to learn as you begin your yoga practice	In sun salutation this pose is done after the upward facing dog pose: - Exhale and lift your hips up - You can keep your knees slightly bent and your heels lifted off the floor - Spread your fingers and press into the thumbs which enables an outward rotation of the upper arms and broadening of the collar bones - Let you head hand and move your shoulder blades away from your ears - Rotate your thighs inwards, push your hips back and sink your heels towards the floor	Checking the position and distance between hands and feet in downward facing dog: - Come into the plank pose - Maintain the same distance between the hands and feet as you push your hips upland back into the downward facing dog pose - Your feet should be hip distance apart. Do not take them too wide (towards the edge of the mat) or too narrow (touching one another)

	- Breath 6 to 15 times - Exhale and come into the next pose which is ashwa sanchalan or otherwise into cat pose	
Starting pose: - Upward facing dog - Cat Pose	- Strengthens the shoulders and the upper body. - Elongates and makes the spine more flexible - Strengthens the hands, wrists, and fingers - Opens up the backs of the legs and the heels - Creates length throughout the body including the heels, calves, hamstrings, hips, glutes, and lower back	- Rejuvenates the entire body - as the heart is higher than your head, it is considered as a mild form of inversion and holds all the benefits of an inversion - Regular practice improves digestion, relieves back pain and helps prevent osteoporosis
Modifications for beginners: - Puppy pose	Contraindications: Do not practice this pose if you	Spiritual awareness: - In the Anahata or the heart

- Downward facing dog with hands on the wall - Downward facing dog with block or bolster under the hands - Downward facing dog with blanket under the heels	have: - Severe carpal tunnel syndrome - Injury to the back, arm or shoulders - High blood pressure - Eye or inner ear infection	chakra - The Vidushi or the throat chakra - The Ajna or the third eye chakra - The uddiyana bandha stimulates the Manipura chakra or the third eye

9. Ashwa Sanchalanasana (Equestrian pose) - same as (4)

10. Hastapadasana (Standing forward bend) - same as (3)

11. Hasta Uttanasana

This is a raised arm pose. It is a standing backbend pose.	- In the standing position or Tadasana, inhale and raise your arms above the head - In a	- In sun salutation, this pose is done smoothly by inhaling and to raise up to Tadasana from

	continuous movement, bend your trunk back slightly to create a simple back bend - Hold the pose for 10 to 15 seconds	hastapadasana or standing forward bend - In the standing position, this pose is done from Tadasana pose
Contraindications: - Some students feel slight pressure on the neck and head when they look down in this pose. They can choose to look up instead - Thai pose should be avoided during pregnancy as the abdominal muscles get compressed	- It helps in the full intake of oxygen. - Expands the chest and ribcage area - Helps keeping the skin firm and healthy - Useful in increasing height	Spiritual awareness: - Anahata Chakra - Vidushi Chakra

12. Tadasana (Mountain Pose)

- Tadasana is also known as mountain pose or samasthiti. It forms a foundation and a prep for other standing poses - it is a starting and	- Stand with both feet slightly apart - Stand evenly on all sides of your feet - Inhale and raise your arms up

finishing pose in the sun salutation series - It is also a resting pose between other strenuous standing poses	- Exhale and raise your shoulders towards your ears - Pay attention to grounding and alignment - Stay still in this position for 6 to 15 breaths - Focus your breathing - Relax and return to the starting position
- The knees should not be locked and you should keep a slight bend in the knees - The thighs and naval center should be gently engaged - When the arms are alongside the body, the palms should be facing outwards to allow for openness across the chest - The chin should be parallel to the floor to create neutral curve in the cervical spine - As a result, the ears, shoulders, hips and ankles should all be in a straight line	As you inhale and raise your arms up there could be variations: - You can interlock your fingers with palms facing up - You can keep your palms slightly apart with fingers facing upwards - You can keep your palms together with fingers facing upwards - In case of neck or shoulder pain, you can look up or look forward or look down
This pose improves - Posture and stability - Gives a sense of focus and grounding - Inner peace as the body and mind is centered - Improves height	Spiritual awareness is on the Muladhara or the root chakra Do not do this pose: - For too long if you have low blood pressure

- instills a sense of confidence	- During pregnancy, keep feet hip distance apart or wider

Chandranamaskar and variations

The moon is our natural satellite. It is associated with many of our pleasant memories, when as children we felt that it followed us everywhere that we went. The moon's light has a soothing effect and when we look at the moon we feel calm and rejuvenated. Moon salutation in hatha yoga shows due respect to the moon as it signifies 'bowing to the moon'.

While Surya Namaskar has 12 poses and steps, Chandranamaskar has 9 poses and 14 steps including prayer positions.

1. Tadasana both hands by your side
2. Inhale and raise your hands up palms together
3. Exhale and bend to the left
4. Come back inhale both hands up
5. Exhale and bend to the right
6. Take left leg to left side to come into a wide legged stance
7. Open your arm shoulder level and inhale
8. Exhale and bend your knees and take both arms into cactus position as you come into the goddess pose then inhale and exhale
9. Adjust your feet with left foot painting towards the left side to enter into trikonasana

10. After that you can choose 2 or 3 asanas like warrior 1 or warrior 2 or parsvottanasana. Any sequence chosen should end with the low lunge extended triangle pose

11. Adjust your feet to come into a half squat on the left side. The right leg will be straight with toes pointing up ; Skandasana, take balance with Namaste mudra

12. Start moving along the ground to the right and bend your right knee to come to malasana. Push both your knees out with your elbows and take a few deep breaths with Namaste mudra

13. Then move towards the right to come into half squat or skandasana on the right side

14. Turn your body towards the right to come into a low lunge in the right side

15. Then do all the earlier asanas in the reverse order, starting with the extended triangle pose and ending with the trikonasana pose.

16. Come all the way up, take a deep breath in and as you exhale squat down into the goddess cactus pose

17. Come back to standing position and bring your right foot in to keep your feet together into mountain pose in Namaste mudra

18. Inhale raise your hand up, keep palms together and exhale bend to the right side and then to the left side and slowly come down to Namaste mudra

19. This was ½ cycle of Chandra namaskar where we move from right to left

20.   Now we will move back from left to right and practice the same sequence

21.   This is one whole cycle of Chandra namaskar

SIVANANDA YOGA

1. Sivananda yoga includes 12 asanas as a system and was named after Guru Sivananda in 1959. This system has since been refined as that of teaching yoga as an exercise, for self-realization, for knowledge of health, peace and unity in diversity.

2. Benefits:
- Good for the energy and Chakra channels
- Good for bones and health

3. Sivananda yoga propagates the practice of selfless service include in karma, dharma, jnana and raja yoga

4. Elements of Sivananda yoga;
- Proper exercise or asanas to enhance the flexibility of joints, muscles, tendons and ligament. To keep the spine strong and flexible for a youthful body
- Proper relaxation or savasana and good sleep to relieve the body and mind from stress and continuous overload
- Proper breathing or pranayama to increase awareness and to overcome depression and stress for better health
- Good diet which is vegetarian including fruits, vegetables, grains, nuts, seeds, legumes and milk
- Positive thoughts and meditation to provide an experience of inner contentment, peace of mind and to live a plausible life

SIVANANDA CLASS - 1 hour 15 minutes

1) Opening **chants**

Dhyana Shlokas

Shanti Mantra

2) Breathing exercises

Kapalabhatti

Anulom Vilom

3) Warm up

Sun Salutation

Leg stretches

Double leg lifts

4) 12 Basic Poses

Inverted sequence

1: Sirshasana - headstand

2: Sarvangasana - shoulder stand

3: Halasana - plough

4: Matsyasana - Fish

Forward & backward bends

5: Paschimottanasana - Sitting Forward Bend

6: Bhujangasana - cobra

7: Salabhasana - locust

8: Dhanurasana - bow

Twists, standing & balancing poses

9: Ardh Matsyendrasana - half Spinal Twist

10: Kakasana - crow

11: Pada hastasana - standing Forward Bend

12: Trikonasana - triangle

5) Relaxation

Final Relaxation

Closing chants
Maha Mrityunjaya Mantras
Peace Mantras

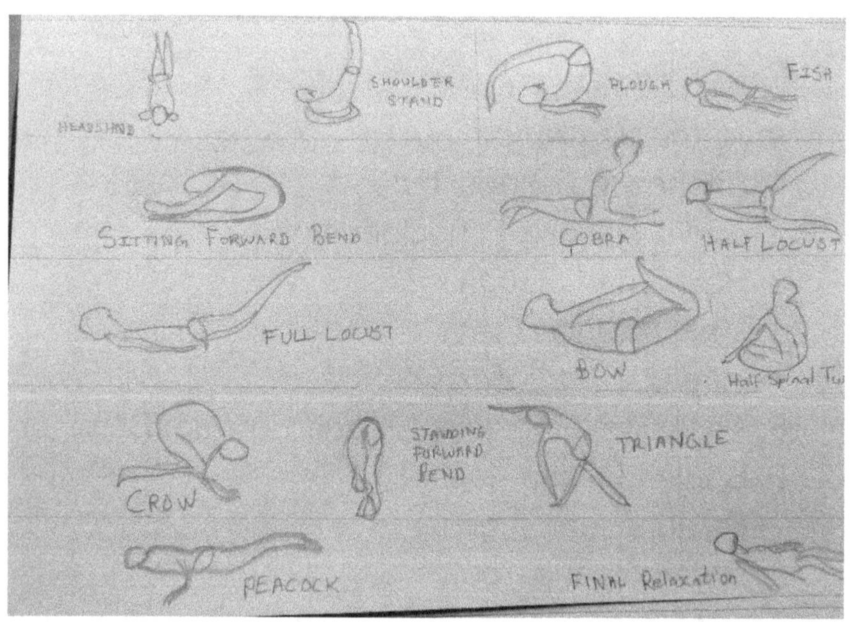

Prenatal and Postnatal Yoga

Why we need to do prenatal yoga -
Prenatal yoga can have a lot of benefits for the practitioner. Prenatal yoga gives strength and energy and pranayama builds lung capacity

CHARACTERISTICS OF PREGNANCY AND PRECAUTIONS TO BE TAKEN:
- During the first 3 months of pregnancy, you have to be very very gentle
- The estimated gestation period is 280 days which is around 42 weeks
- At 37 weeks the baby is fully developed
- At 40 weeks pregnancy the pregnancy is completed
- During the pregnancy there are 3 trimesters. The total gestation time is 3*3 months which is nine months
- During the FIRST TRIMESTER PLEASE AVOID YOGA PRACTICE. This is because it is a complicated time where there is vomiting and many changes are happening within the body. In case of miscarriage they will directly blame the yoga teacher
- During the FIRST TRIMESTER practice only simple inhalation and simply exhalation

- There are different asanas during that can be practiced during each trimester to give different kinds of strength and flexibility
- During pregnancy, everyday changes happen within the body. Look for ahimsa or nonviolence which is not to hurt yourself
- As the baby grows it changes position. So your practice always depends on your health and the position of the baby. You should not force yourself to do yoga practice. Many changes have happened inside the body and so your practice will vary according to the situation of the body.

For the yoga teachers:

- Find out some things for prenatal health and yoga and then make the course

- Know how to design the right practice for each student

Prenatal yoga is not about women sacrificing their bodies for the good of the baby. Instead it is an honoring of the union between mother and baby. Preparing a mothers' body to be strong and flexible so that she and her baby can work together in pregnancy and childbirth to have a gentle and empowering birth experience.

Prenatal yoga: how a pregnant body works and how to modify poses for individual needs
Pregnancy consists of 3 trimesters, each about 3 months long. In each trimester there are specific poses that are beneficial for the pregnant body, to

reduce discomfort and to strengthen the body in preparation for labor and childbirth. Some days a certain pose may feel wonderful and on other days it may not feel good at all. The most important aspect of prenatal yoga is one that is practiced in all yoga, which is ahimsa or non-violence towards yourself and others. This means allowing the body to only do poses that feel good. This is more important in prenatal yoga as the baby grows and changes position often. There are times when a certain pose may not be conducive to the position of the baby. Forcing positions in order to repeat them is inappropriate for pregnant women and can cause strain.

How prenatal yoga helps

1. The focus and connection with breath. Yoga can increase lung capacity allowing the woman to take deeper longer breaths, which bring more oxygen to the baby and mom, making contractions feel shorter and more manageable.
2. Women who do prenatal yoga have more stamina as their prenatal yoga practice builds strength and flexibility while staying focused on the breath while releasing tension. They can go a longer time without pain medications.
3. Prenatal yoga releases endorphins or the feel good hormones, which she becomes accustomed to feeling while practicing yoga. The same hormones are released in labor and are identifiable to women who have been practicing yoga.

4. Practicing relaxation at the end of class helps women get familiar with what their bodies feel like when they are comfortable and free of tension. It also gives them a practice of staying in the moment and focused.

For information only

Tests
First trimester
- Blood type and Rh factor
- Anemia
- Blood test or CBC for hemoglobin, hematocrit and platelet count
- Hepatitis B, Syphilis, and HIV.
- Immunity to German measles (rubella) and chickenpox (varicella)
- Cystic fibrosis and spinal muscular atrophy

Second trimester
- Weight
- Blood pressure
- Urine test for bacteria, protein or sugar
- Baby's heartbeat
- Measuring the height of the uterus to track the baby's growth and position
- Ultrasound fetal anomaly scan to check the baby's organs, structure and growth and establish the gestational age and size

Third trimester
- Screening test for Down's syndrome, Edward's syndrome and Patau's syndrome to

assess the chances of the baby having one of these conditions

Changing body

First trimester

- Feeling more tired than usual
- Need to urinate more often
- Painful breasts and morning sickness
- Heartburn and faster heart rates because the body produces more blood to support the baby

Second trimester

- The symptoms of the first trimester start to subside
- Heart stills pumps fast and may cause dizziness
- The extra blood may cause nose bleeds and bleeding gums
- Constipation and back pain may develop
- A baby bump begin to develop

Third trimester:

- Increased skin temperature as the fetus radiates body heat, causing the mother to feel hot
- Need to urinate more often because of increased pressure on the bladder
- Swelling of the ankles, hands, and face (edema) due to retention of fluids

Baby's Development

- First trimester: The baby will grow from a fertilized egg into a moving fetus with eyes, ears, and working organs
- Second trimester: The baby's features develop and you may be able to feel your baby move
- Third trimester: The baby's bones will harden and will open and close their eyes. The baby grows rapidly and positions head down to get ready for birth

The three layers of the uterus

- Perimetrium: The outermost, protective layer of the uterus
- Myometrium: The highly muscular middle layer which expands during pregnancy and contracts to push your baby out
- Endometrium: The inner layer or lining of the uterus; the uterine lining

Pregnancy hormones

- The main hormones are estrogen and progesterone
- The woman will produce more estrogen during 1 pregnancy than her entire life
- The increase in estrogen during pregnancy helps a woman produce increased blood vessels or vascularization
- Progesterone helps the uterine lining to become receptive to implantation of a fertilized egg
- Progesterone and relaxin help soften ligaments and cartilage and loosen the joints to prepare for childbirth

- The other main pregnancy hormones that have a role to bring changes within the uterus and the whole body include:

  - FSH (follicle stimulating hormone)

  - LH (luteinizing hormone)

  - HCG (human chorionic gonadotropin)

  - Relaxin

  - Placental growth factor

  - HPL (human placental lactogen)

  - Oxytocin

  - Prolactin

Baby positions

It is helpful to know the position of the baby near the end of pregnancy as optimal fetal position can reduce the length of labor and pushing and increase the comfort of the mother. Yoga and movement can help achieve this optimal positioning especially if the mother knows the position of the baby before labor begins.

Baby positions

Babies have plenty of room to move around prior to about 34 weeks. Therefore, the position of the baby can change often prior to that.

Yoga movements that assist in correcting less than optimal positioning

Prenatal Yoga Routine

The Don'ts
Do not compress stomach
Do not sit on block

The Do's
- Decide the level of practice. This is decided according to the practice level of the student
- The student can use mat, blanket or towel
- Mindfulness meditation can be taken up. The student can sit on the pillow

Practice during the 2nd and 3rd trimesters
Very very slow and gentle practice (every yoga practice start and end with relaxation)

Sitting asana practice:
1. Relaxation ie- 5, with chi mudra or namaste mudra omkar palming
2. Head rotations
3. Open arms shoulder level - both hands up and down- 2
4. Hands behind back- lift your shoulders -drop shoulders -look up - palm on the knees- suck your belly look down
5. Sideways bending 2
6. Both hands up fingerlock - look up
7. Both Legs Straight- relax your leg move your leg - alternate foot flexing
8. Butterfly- press your knees down

9. Shoulders up and down

10. Palms on the knees - Chakki chalasana

11. Both hands up look up - palms on the knees look down - 2-4 times

12. Sideways bending

13. Sideways twisting

14. Legs straight a little apart from each other - hands more behind back - relax your legs and move your legs- move your knees up and down - rotation

15. Gentle butterfly - knees up and down. This practice is very good for normal delivery

Breathing

- Breathing is a most important practice
- Breathing also calms fears and pain
- Fears and pain can make us hold our breath
- Connection within ourselves
- Helps during childbirth as the connection between movement and breath during labor time   can release pain and fear :   the correlation is too great to ignore or just write off as a correlation
- Breath = life

PRACTICE 1

- **Gentle Cat Cow** is a good pregnancy routine. It should be done with gentle alignment - 4 times
- To maintain the gap between the hands and the knees, hold opposite elbow and adjust the gap
- Shoulder and wrist should be aligned
- Shoulder should be away from the ear

- Knee to hip distance comes naturally depends on the length of the hip
- inhale - push your hip up- do only as much as you want and do not strain your neck muscles
- Exhale - just look down - do not compress your belly
- They can relax in Vajrasana or Virasana

PRACTICE 2
- **Cat - only single leg** stretched back straight out (do not bring your hand forward)
- **Cat - only single leg** straight back and then leg sidewise which is called as the Tiger pose
- The student can lift her leg up or keep her leg on the mat. This depends on the practice level of the student and so the position in which she is feeling comfortable

PRACTICE 3
- **Cat - only single leg** straight back and then step by step bring leg sideways with the support of the ground

- Practice 2 and 3 are done on both sides. After sufficient practice. all these three practices can be held for 6 - 10 counts - this will bring the strength and movement flexibility will improve

PRACTICE 4
- **Cat - only single hand and single leg** straight forward and backwards. The students can practice the same things we did before in practice 2 and 3. However, do not bring them

directly to this practice as it can strain the body. The teacher should decide the level of practice according to the practice level of the student

Prenatal guidelines for teachers a 45 minutes class sequence

The student can practice one asana at a time for 3-4 times. In the second time let them hold the asana for 7-10 counts, so that their strength and energy levels can be increased. The practitioner can sit on a chair for the sitting sequence

- Deep and relaxed breathing , omkara, palming
- Very relaxed opening exercises - flexing one foot at a time
- Music and Meditation for ½ an hour or 45 minutes
- Seated exercises for the head and shoulders movements
- Fingerlock in front and stretch both arms in frontside - 5-10 times
- Fingerlock and take both hands upside then bring both hands down for 5 - 10 times. The student can also practice with a strap or towel
- Put hands behind hips and lift the spine up
- Modified practice in prenatal yoga - you can drop the elbow on the knee - sideways bending. This will create space in torso when the arms are lifted for a side bend or in a backbend

Action and Homework for the Teachers

- Make the classes into **3-4 batches** in order to take the asana practice systematically to build up strength and flexibility.
- The first is **the basic batch** consisting of simple meditation, pranayama and sitting asana practice
- You can tell the students that after you finish this batch **then the next batch starts**. Start the cat- cow and all the cat routines step by step
- Don't just give directions. Also get involved with the effectiveness of the practice.
- Give clear directions when giving yoga practice
- Voice should be very deep and humble when giving relaxation practice. The voice modulation of the teacher is a very important part of teaching
- Write down your sequences for the classes
- If you find something more than what is given in this manual, then you add it to the class according to your understanding
- Make your own assessment from time to time by getting feedback from the students and also give feedback and suggestions to yourself. This can improve the quality and effectiveness of your class

Postnatal Yoga

- Postnatal yoga is recommended to be practiced after 6 weeks of normal delivery and longer after a cesarean
- As the body has undergone many changes that you had 9 months back, you will need to start slowly, listen to your body and adapt poses as needed
- As with the prenatal yoga practice, ease yourself back into the yoga routine and be gentle with yourself. New mothers who are breastfeeding may be uncomfortable lying on their stomach or do other poses that involve the knees, chest and chin
- So the post-natal classes have to be modified and some poses have to be substituted

Some sample post-natal classes for the first weeks of practice:

The warm - up sequence:
1. Sukhasana or siddhasana and head rotations: This helps to sit comfortably and easily with a straight back and reduce stiffness moving through the areas of tightness in the neck
2. Eagle arms; arms crossed, bent, and parallel to the floor
3. Easy twist and forward bending

Lying down with the back and practice the following exercises
1) Pelvic tilts: Lying down on the mat; bring the back firmly on to the mat. Open your arms at shoulder level and gently move your pelvis

side to side. It is a subtle stretch that reduces stiffness and helps warm up the spine.
2) Single leg lifts: It helps in regaining strength in the leg and to stretch the hamstrings, feet, shins and calves
3) Lying down pigeon or eye of the needle pose

Cat - cow
1. Cat cow stretch
2. Needle the thread pose; sucirandhrasana

Downward facing dog
1. Walk your heels up and down
2. Gently dip shoulders and feel the stretch

Child's pose keeping pillow or cushion under the shoulders and chest
1. Stretch your arms and stretch your spine
2. Needle the thread

Goddess pose
1. Eagle arms
2. Arms up and down
3. Gently bend and straighten your knees

Stretches for nursing mothers
- Cow -cat
- Sphinx
- Heart opening with a bolster or a block
- Bridge pose - Setu Bandhasana
- Shoulder stand - Sarvangasana
- Half boat pose - Parsva Navasana
- Forward fold with fingerlock behind back
- Extended triangle - Utthita Trikonasana

- Downward Facing Dog - Adho Mukha Svanasana

The six best poses after delivery and after a few weeks regular practice are

- Cat and cow pose
- Plank pose
- Revolved triangle pose
- Malasana
- Hanumanasana

Standing sequence after a few weeks regular practice

1. Downward Facing Dog
2. High lunge with variations
3. Warrior 1, 2 and reverse warrior
4. Extended side angle pose - utthita parsvakonasana with variations
5. Extended triangle - Utthita Trikonasana
6. Half-moon - Ardha chandrasana
7. Downward facing dog, adho mukha svanasana

Sitting sequence after a few weeks regular practice
- Sukhasana or siddhasana
- Side bending
- Side twisting
- Forward bending
- Both hands behind back - bend back
- Naukasana
- Bend knees - both hands behind back - walk your hands back
- Open one leg sideways - side bending twisting, gentle forward and back bend

- Sitting side split - Side bending and twisting - gentle forward and back bending

Core exercises after a few weeks regular practice
- Standing _ Twisting, konasana 2, leg kick ups, touching opposite side toes
- Sitting - Naukasana, elbows down - single and both leg lifts, single and both legs cycling, single and both legs rotation
- Lying down - Setu Bandhasana pulses, Single leg crunches, both legs up crunches, single leg lifts, sideways leg lifts

A daily routine for regular practitioners:
1. Pelvic tilts
2. Cat cow stretch
3. Downward facing dog
4. Low lunges
5. Straight leg lunge - Parsvottanasana
6. Tadasana - Uttanasana
7. Standing forward bend - Pada hastasana
8. Downward dog to pigeon pose
9. Happy baby pose
10. Spinal twist
11. Savasana
12. If you are feeling energetic, then you can practice to improve on your headstand, bakasana and so on

Guidelines for Beginners

Timings

Yoga is best practiced in the morning between 5 to 6 am on an empty stomach

Yoga can be practiced in the afternoon. However don't have a meal or coffee or tea 21/2 to 3 hours before the practice

A relatively empty and quiet place should be chosen for yoga practice

Yoga is better practiced on a yoga mat or on a carpet rather than on the bare floor

Practice

Practice 60 minutes of yoga and meditation with breathing every day, you will start getting good results very soon

Patience is important for your practice

Keep a flexible schedule and keep practicing continuously. This habit will keep you healthy, happy and you get the results that you expect

Air

It's good to practice in the fresh air. Ensure that there is proper ventilation by keeping the windows open

It is not advisable to put on the air conditioner or the fan whilst practicing yoga. Switch off air conditioner and fan while practicing

Yoga can be done in an open place also

Energy

While doing meditation, you can cover yourself with a blanket or bed sheet

While practicing asana, pranayama and/or meditation, the body will release a lot of energy. This energy helps heals the immune system, regulates the breathing pattern, helps calm the mind and experience peace

Silence

Maintain silence while doing yoga practice

Do not talk and try to focus on your practice

Switch off the TV and mobile phones whilst practicing

Liquid
- Yoga should not be practiced immediately after drinking coffee or tea

    You should have gap of 21/2 hours after drinking any drink

Water
  - Right after yoga practice should not drink water
  - The exceptional circumstance is emergency
  - After a minimum of 30.mins to an hour, you can drink water at room temperature
  - Don't drink cold water because it will increase any existing pain in your body and create other difficulties

Number of times

  - Yoga is normally practiced once a day
  - In case of some problems or disease then you can practice yoga twice a day as it gives better results

Awareness
  - During the yoga practice you should have full attention concentration and Awareness
  - Whenever you feel pressure, stretch or pain, you should take your awareness to that place. It enables better and faster relief and de stress. The practice becomes more effective

Reactions
  - Try not to give negative reactions to pain or stretch as you advance into your yoga practice
  - First accept that pain and then treat it by just doing yoga to the extent that your body allows you
  - Negative reactions can increase the pain and will not solve the pain and stretch

Abilities
  - While doing yoga practice, observe your abilities and do the practice a accordingly

- In the beginning we feel the body pain starting or increasing. This is because the body is not used the muscles and joints opening up in the yoga practice and hence you feel that pain
- Have turmeric and pepper to improve your bone health
- During the first week of practice, if you have pain in your body, you can drink one cup of milk before going to sleep. You can also mix 1 tablespoon of haldi into the drink. If you don't have diabetes you can also add sugar

Thinking

- While practicing yoga you should have positive thinking
- It will take you on the way towards excellent results from yoga

Painkillers

- Painkillers may cure the symptoms, but may not eradicate the cause of the pain on a longer term. Yoga helps to take the pain out from its root cause

Mind

- When you are practicing the asanas, put you whole attention into it
- Don't take your mind into the past or into the future to make plans

Rest

- While practicing asanas, In the beginning keep the eyes open and when you feel more

comfortable in the pose and are holding the pose for a longer time, then close the eyes
- If you cannot do yoga in the standing position then you can take the help of wall

Prana
- In most of the yoga practice, keep regular and normal breathing
- Do not hold the breath unless and until guided

Regularity
- Continuous yoga practice is necessary for better results
- You can plan it according to the time available so that you find it possible to practice

Vata and Kapha
- Air or vata when it is imbalanced can cause a lot of pain in the body
- Kapha brings heaviness
- Avoid vata from foods like rice, yogurt banana, beans etc. before going to bed

Action and Relaxation
- After every yoga action there must be relaxation in the form of savasana
- This helps you to reap the benefits of your practice and gives higher and better results

Stamina
- You can increase the speed of the practice slowly
- Increase the time of the practice gradually

- For the first week start with 40 minutes next week 50 minutes and then go for 60 minutes
- This practice will build up stamina

Imbalance in the energy causes imbalance in the body and the mind. So you should be aware of some things about your body and your yoga practice.

Body pain best practices:
If you are suffering from knee or back pain then perform yogic jogging slowly.
The yoga practitioner can also use some pillows, blankets and blocks in their yoga practice.
They should not give pressure or strain to the affected area.
If a person cannot practice yoga in the standing position then they can do it in sitting position. Otherwise you can also practice in the lying down position
If you still have other problems, then contact your doctor

Recommended habits:
In the morning when you wake up take warm water instead of tea
If you are suffering from constipation, you can take amla juice in hot water
In the beginning days of yoga practice, take hot milk with turmeric

Best practices for sleeping
While lying down on the back, bring awareness on your breath and leave your whole body loose it will

reduce thoughts and you will have deeper and better sleep

Before going to sleep, leave all the tensions behind and say to yourself that ' when I wake up, only then I will deal with them'

Too many thoughts you are trying to control the future, but in the reality no one can control the future

Asana best practices

Normally you should know that yoga is not only about the flexibility

Simple poses done with more awareness then they can give you better results

If you want to master asanas you will hold the pose for a long time

Asana is a journey from outside to inside

And then to full of awareness of total fitness of body mind

An effortless pose coming from infinity is called mastery of asana

WHAT TO TEACH NEW YOGA STUDENTS

OUTLINE OF THE TEACHING SEQUENCES:

- The sequences should invariably include twisting
- The single series poses can be repeated. Each pose can be taken up 2-3 times with 5 or 10 breaths
- The class should include pranayama and mudras; a combination of both
- The class should end with meditation and shavasana
- The class can end with lotus mudra

STANDARD POSES FOR REGULAR PRACTICE:

STANDING POSES:
- **Tadasana** can be practiced for 5 repetitions for 5 breaths each cycle
- **Kati Chakrasana** is a twisting pose and is to be practiced from both sides with normal breathing. You can take repetitions of up to 10 rounds with holding for six breaths at the end of the repetitions.
- **Trikonasana** or triangle pose can be repeated 2 times continuously to hold with 10 breaths
- **Padahastasana** is a standing forward fold and is to be practiced with knees bent or knees straight. Regular practice may be necessary before the students becomes more familiar and flexible in the pose. To repeat

Padahastasana, you may like to choose a transitory pose like utkatsana or half forward fold with or without holding, according to the requirement of the students.

SITTING POSES:
Choose a continuous and effective sequence in the sitting poses. Each pose may be practiced up to 5 to 10 times depending on the theme of your class; whether its flexibility of weight loss or strength. Each pose can be practiced with 5 to 6 breaths holds or practiced continuously with breath holds at the final round.

- Chakki Chalasana may be done sitting cross legged or with legs opened sideways. This sitting forward rotations with interlocked fingers or a fist, builds up core strength and flexibility
- Vajrasana pose is not a beginner's pose and may be done by sitting on 1 or 2 blocks. The students may be given regular practice to gain more flexibility
- Virasana or hero's pose also may be done step by step. A block or pillow may be placed under back initially for support. Regular practice may be required for strength and flexibility for the pose
- Animal pose with twisting, side bending and forward bending variations
- Cat cow may be done continuously with instructions
- Lying down on the wheel. Here the student may need support for the back and/or the wheel, by the teacher or fellow students

- Legs straight, relax your legs move your legs. The variations in this pose are sideways twisting, paschimmotanasana and purvatasana
- Elbow Lock under knees - knee bending - knees rotation
- Pulling the rope or rajju karshasana
- Boating pose or navasana
- Half butterfly pose or Janu Sirshasana
- Half lotus pose or ardh baddha paschimmotanasana or ardh padmasana
- Heron pose or krounchaasana
- Single leg boat or naukasana
- Ek pada sirhasana preparation poses
- Ek pada koundinasana preparation poses
- Paschimottanasana or forward bending pose
- Shashankasana (child pose) - frog pose
- Vakrasana
- Ardh matsyendrasana

PRONE POSES:
Each pose may be done 2 - 3 times. Each pose may be done for 1 to 2 minutes

- Bhujangasana
- Ardha salabhasana- raise one leg up
- Dhanurasana (bow pose)
- Yastikasana (stick pose)
- Viparita salabhasana or superman pose with variations

SUPINE POSES:
Each pose may be done 2 - 3 times. Each pose may be done for 1 to 2 minutes

- Pawanmuktasana
- Setu Bandhasana
- Supta Baddhakonasana
- Single leg crunches
- Yogic cycling
- Yogic leg rotation
- Sideways leg lifts
- Shoulder stand prep

Cooling practices

- Sideways twisting - lying down on the belly or lying down on the back - all variations
- Anulom vilom pranayama: 5 – 10 times
- Bhramari pranayama: 5 -10 times
- Meditation for 5 to 20 minutes

Opening and closing poses may consist of

- Omkara and relaxation
- Some simple basic side stretches in easy sitting pose
- Baddhakonasa with variations
- Open legs sideways - all variations

MUDRAS

These mudras may be added them into the personalized yoga routine

- Brahma mudra	- Nadanusandhana Pranayama (Pranayama with sound) with Chi, Chinmaya, Adi and Merudanda or Brahma mudra	
- Hasta	- Jyana	
- Yoga	- Varun	
- Shunya	- Surya	
- Apana	- Sanjeevani	
- Linga	- Majasir	
- Hakini	- Saman	
- Bhairav	- Hyidya	
	-	

MANTRAS

Mantra at the beginning of the class:

Om sahana bhavatu
Sahanau bhunaktu
Saha viryam karva vahi
Tejas vinaa
Vadhitamastu
Maa vidhwisha vahai
Om shanti shanti shanti

Mantra	Meaning of this shloka or prayer
	Oh lord protect all of

	us
Om sahana bhavatu	Oh lord protect all of us
Sahanau bhunaktu	And help us that we get the capacity to study and understand
Saha viryam karva vahi	We acquired the knowledge
Tejas vinaa	With the acquisition of this knowledge let peace flow in us
Vadhitamastu	And help us that we get brilliant
Maa vidhwisha vahai	We don't hold any enmity against anyone
Om shanti shanti shanti	Om peace peace peace

After chanting
Eyes closed rub your palms and place them over your eyes
Feel the heat of your palms over your eyes and take this energy in. Bend a little forward. Then, slowly come back and gently open your eyes.

Mantra after the class:
After all yoga practices close your eyes and chant this shloka after Om chanting

Om sarve bhavantu sukhina
Sarve santu niravanamaya
Sarve bhadrani paschyantu
Maa kaschif dukh bhag bhavej
Om shanti shanti shanti

Mantra	Meaning
Om sarve bhavantu sukhina	Oh lord may all be happy
Sarve santu niravanamaya	May all be free from disease
Sarve bhadrani paschyantu	May all have peace and happiness in their life
Maa kaschif dukh bhag bhavej	No one suffers from sorrows
Om shanti shanti shanti	Om peace peace peace

One more prayer

Om asato maa sadgamaya
Tomaso maa jyotiram gamaya
Mrytonma amritam gamaya
Om shanti shanti shanti

Mantra	Meaning
Om asato maa	Lead me from the

sadgamaya	unreal to the real
Tomaso maa jyotiram gamaya	From darkness to light
Mrytonma amritam gamaya	From death to immortality
Om shanti shanti shanti	Om peace peace peace

A MODEL CLASS

1. Sitting position

Knee bending

Chakki chalasana or sitting twisting

Malasana or garland pose

2. Core Asanas

Cow cat straight led and straight hand 5 times to hold each side

Cow cat needle the thread

3. Prone position

Bhujangasana to child 1 time or 3 times to hold

Lying down with the chest - drop leg other side

4. Sitting position

1 sequence in the sitting position:

Paschimottanasana- heron - janu sirshasana - ardh matsyendrasana

5. Power, flexibility, core and weight loss flow

Cow cat- low lunge - high lunge – warrior 2 - parsvottanasana or pyramid pose– pigeon pose – vakrasana

6. More core poses

Downward facing dog - Knee to nose

7. Lying down with the chest

Dhanurasana - single leg dhanurasana
Lying down with the chest - bend knee sideways –
relax

8. Lying down with the back
Other standard core exercises: Hand behind head
raise your head and chest as in reverse crunches -
raise your legs up as in leg lifts- Cactus position-
raise your head and chest and legs up as in
naukasana boat pose

Pranayama Practice
Yogic breathing
Mahabandha
Anulom vilom pranayama followed with jalandhara
bandha
Shitkari pranayama
Chandra Bhedana
Bhramari

Meditation and savasana

SOME POSTURES ALIGNMENT AND MODIFICATIONS

Here are some examples of how you may teach the postures alignment and modifications to your students.

1) TADASANA- palm tree pose

- Keep the chest front side
- Shoulder drawn behind the chest
- Arms are aligned away from the ears
- Pelvic position is in the front tilt
- Pada Bandha may be assumed to stabilize the foot
- Relax the shoulders
- Try and keep the legs straight

The upper body affects the lower body and so we have to bring their connection. These same rules apply to all other standing postures. Observe with awareness about how the whole body is engaged and how the inner thigh is engaged

Modifications

- Both hands behind back
- Finger lock behind the neck
- Both hands by side
- Both hands up with palms together or finger lock

- These can also be practiced with the strap or towel
- For lower body modifications, raise the heels
- You can stand on the block
- You can practice with the support of the wall
- Feet together or feet a little apart
- Modifications are based on the practice and also the type of students (for example if the student with shoulder pain then keep the hands by side of body ; if any student with knee or ankle pain then there no need to stand on heels, for frozen shoulders you can give practice with strap or towel)

TIRYAKA TADASANA

- Tadasana combined with side movement
- You just have to control the lateral movement
- There is no back tilt only front pelvic tilt
- Assume padam bandha
- Lower body is stabilized and only upper body is moved. As the hips are not moved, this also avoids the hyper movement

Modifications
- Both hands up with palms together or finger lock
- Both hands behind neck with finger lock
- Hands on waist
- One hand behind back the other hand extended up
- One hand on waist the other hand extended up
- Ardhakati chakrasana

- Both hands up parallel with palms not together
- Elbow lock
- Feet together or feet apart

Breathing -
- Yogic breathing – The duration depends on different body types and different breath capacities
Example: for 10 counts you can take 5 - 10 breaths
Breathing should be continuous- never hold the breath (except in certain asanas like mandukasana or bandhas)
- By understanding these concepts, the yoga instructor may change their personal approach to teach their students

Question Paper

Every moment of our life is an outcome of not only our birth and circumstances but also of our experience and knowledge. You can ask yourself whether a 'life exam' is important or is just a written exam for a course.

In a 'life exam' the more we are ourselves, the better are the results of the 'exam'. With bliss within oneself; the examination of life is successfully passed. If in the current moment, we are tense, the next moment will also be tense. Current moment sows the seed for the next moment. These moments added together become life. Life's exam teaches us to live mindfully without any effort and with ease in the present moment, to live our lives without any worries, stresses and tensions.

When we 'spend' time on browsing the internet without an objective, it reduces the time that we have. However, when we 'spend' time on knowledge, it increases our experience and teaching capacity. A written exam is akin to 'spending' time on one's knowledge. This is because knowledge increases by studying, learning and then giving exams. An exam in the knowledge of yoga is not a competitive exam. It is rather a process of gaining self-knowledge, finding new aspects within oneself and is refining and purifying oneself. An exam in Yoga is to ensure that when you complete it, you will naturally guide/teach/help others as you become self-inspired and self-sufficient in knowledge and communication.

Yoga leads us to cultivate a calm and steady mind. Yoga exams are necessary to ensure that you can impart your wisdom and knowledge to your students. It also serves to give feedback to your teachers about their learning and teaching knowledge and whether it has been practical and effective.

You don't need to be panicky, serious or worried. Just be calm, have a grounded/steady mind by being regular with your Yoga classes. Be sincere with your learning to prepare yourself for success. Your sincerity and genuineness will first benefit YOU.

According to the Bhagavad-Gita, one should keep striving and working towards one's objective without wondering about the fruits of one's labor. Being joyous and happy makes you pass life's exam and gives you blissful results in your written exam as well!!

Wishing you blissful learning and all the best!!

Kavita Sinha

Topics covered in the exam:

1. Pranayama

- What is pranayama
- Tell all the names and types of pranayama
- What is puraka rechaka and kumbhaka?
- Tell about nadis; the ida pingala and sushumna nadis
- Know about each pranayama
- The benefits of each pranayama
- Who should and should not do certain pranayama
- What are the different types of breathing

Bandhas
- How many bandhas are there? Name them

Chakras
- What are chakras
- Position name and color of the chakras

Mudras

- Why we use mudras
- What are their benefits
- How many types of mudras are there
- What is the relation between the five elements and the five fingers
- Tell the name of any 6 mudras

Shatkarmas

- What are the different types of Shatkarmas
- Name the Shatkarmas

Prayers and Mantras

- What are mantras
- What are prayers
- Why we chant mantras and do prayers
- Should know how to chant and how to write

Yoga Teacher

- What are the potent qualities of a yoga teacher
- What are the guidelines for a yoga teacher and for a beginner; the person who is starting yoga for the first time

Yoga Nidra and Meditation

- What are they
- How to do them

Types of yoga

- Sivananda
- Astanga
- Hatha
- Power
- Prenatal yoga
- Know the sequences for all of these

Practical things

- How to teach asana
- How to teach relaxation
- How to talk
- Also should know about the sequences - sitting and standing positions
- Types of postures in hip opening and back bend class
- Prayers and pranayama you should know how to teach

Know how to teach different types of yoga

- With ball
- With chair
- Stick yoga
- With strap
- With block
- Sitting
- Standing

Conclusion:

This book is meant to serve a guide for yoga teachers who are imparting yoga teacher training to their students. This book is to be used for YTTC 200 hours and 300 hours and 500 hours; according to how you. The teacher, plans your course. This book can be used as a guide in any country for imparting training to yoga students. Do get in touch with me in the event that you have any queries via my email

kavi@yogayouandfitness.com.

Wish you the best in your endeavors!!

Kavita Sinha